The Easy 5-Ingredient
Healthy Cookbook

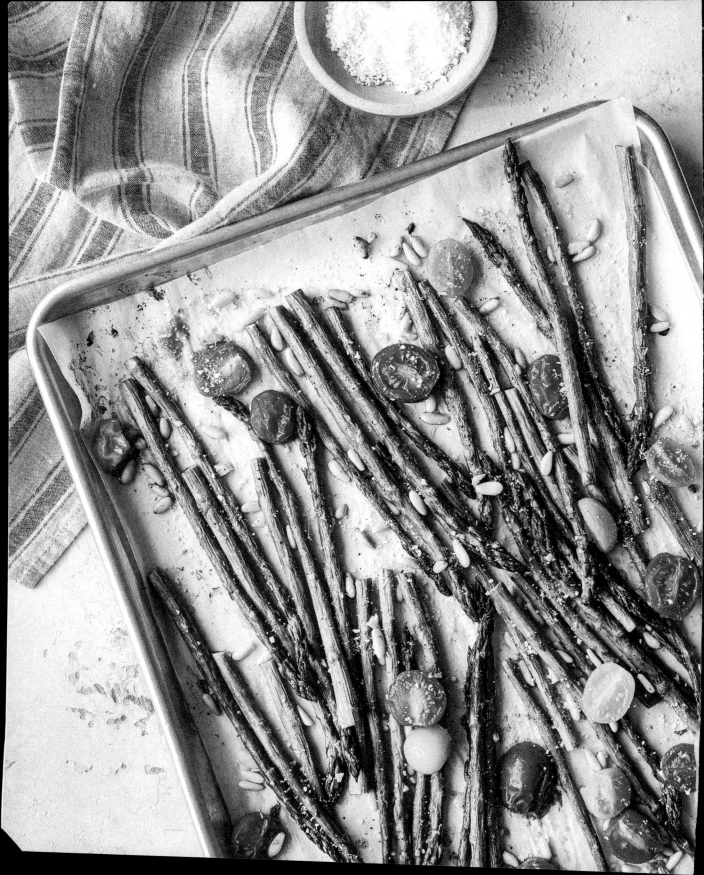

The Easy
5-INGREDIENT
HEALTHY COOKBOOK

Simple Recipes to Make Healthy Eating Delicious

Toby Amidor, MS, RD, CDN

Photography by Hélène Dujardin

ROCKRIDGE
PRESS

For general information on our other products and services or to obtain technical support, please contact our Customer Care Department within the United States at (866) 744-2665, or outside the United States at (510) 253-0500.

Rockridge Press publishes its books in a variety of electronic and print formats. Some content that appears in print may not be available in electronic books, and vice versa.

Photography © Hélène Dujardin, Food styling by Tami Hardeman

ISBN: Print 978-1-64152-004-1 | eBook 978-1-64152-005-8

To my amazing children,
Schoen, Ellena, and Micah.
You are the lights of my life and
my motivation for everything
I accomplish. I love you.

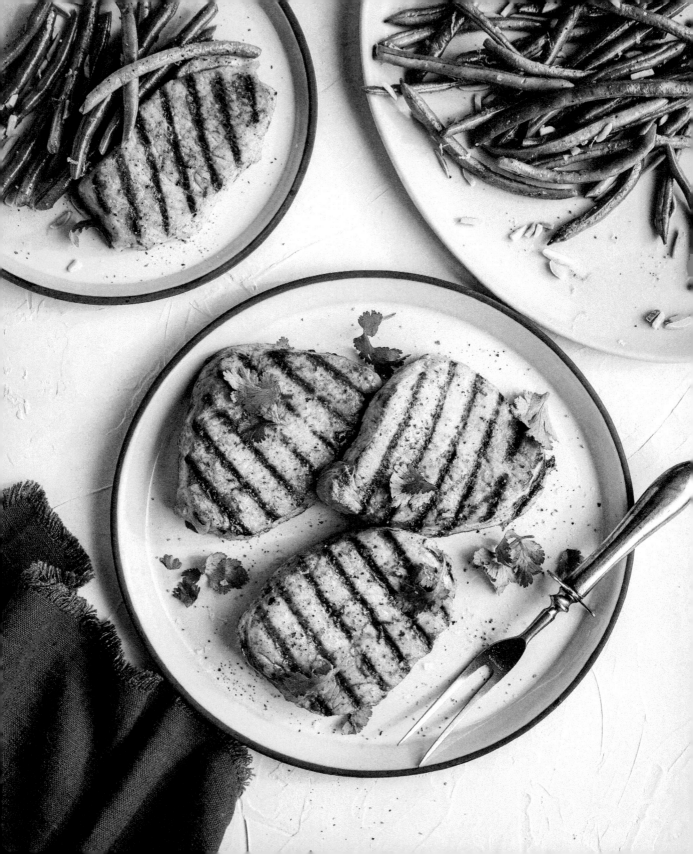

Contents

Introduction

One of the most precious commodities you have is time. How often have you wished for 25 hours in a day? Unfortunately, you can't extend the time in a day, but you can cut back on certain things that waste your precious time. Although it's necessary to be in the kitchen to cook and prepare delicious meals, you don't have to slave over a hot stove for hours. You can make simple, healthy, delicious meals with five or fewer ingredients and get in and out of the kitchen in no time and back to your life.

At the age of 32, I had three kids under five years old. With my third child, I was back to work the same day I came home from the hospital. I remember working on my computer, rocking my daughter in her car seat with my feet while I typed on my keyboard. At the time, I was the director of nutrition at a startup online wellness company. In between rocking my daughter, I also had to pick up my son at nursery school and make sure everyone was fed. With three young kids and a full-time job, my meals *had* to be quick and easy. I planned dishes that I could whip up with an ingredient list that didn't break the bank and consisted of easy-to-find foods. I found the perfect balance between saving time and providing healthy meals for me and my family. I'll admit, I thought I was a genius and patted myself on the back a few times (probably because I was so sleep deprived), but the point is this: Even if you're sleep deprived and stretched to the max, you don't have to live on bagel bites, chicken nuggets, and prepared frozen meals. With the same amount of effort, you can enjoy real, whole-food meals—and I'll show you how.

Although creating five-ingredient recipes isn't a new concept, it's become more popular than ever due to the increased hustle and bustle of everyday life. In my second cookbook, *The Healthy Meal Prep Cookbook*, I explain how to manage your time by planning and preparing several dishes over the weekend to have on hand for the busy workweek ahead. Between creating healthy five-ingredient meals and managing meal prep, you can slam-dunk that time crunch that stresses most people out!

This cookbook contains over 150 healthy five-ingredient recipes. Think of them as building blocks, or the most basic form, of the recipe—you can build on them over time. Throughout this cookbook, I will provide actionable tips for almost every recipe, labeled Toby's Tip, on how to swap alternative ingredients or add in ingredients so you can individualize the dish to please your palate. Toby's Tip may also be a quick culinary trick that has worked for me in the kitchen and that I hope works for you as well. For example, I don't want to spend extra money purchasing low-sodium canned beans, and you shouldn't have to, either. Studies have found that rinsing your canned beans under cool running water can reduce the amount of sodium by up to 40 percent! It is these types of "aha" tips that you will find in almost every recipe.

Throughout the first chapter, you'll discover tips and tricks to make healthy cooking easier. I'll offer quick and easy shortcuts, like preparing and storing ingredients ahead of time, bulk cooking, and repurposing leftovers into a whole new dish. I'll tell you which seven ingredients you should have in your pantry at all times, share some simple guidelines for "clean eating," and tell you what's in season throughout the year.

All of the recipes in this cookbook were carefully selected based on four criteria: They are easy to prepare, call for easy-to-find ingredients, keep nutrition in mind, and taste delicious. As such, most of these recipes are one-pot (or one-pan) meals, can be prepared in 30 minutes or less, use a slow cooker, or are freezer friendly. Each recipe is also labeled for special eating preferences, including Gluten-Free, Dairy-Free, Paleo-Friendly, Vegan, and Vegetarian. I also provide a nutrition breakdown for each recipe, including calories, total fat, saturated fat, protein, carbohydrates, fiber, and sodium. My recipes always specify the exact serving size (portion), such as how many cups of pasta or tablespoons of dressing correspond to the nutrition numbers. That way, if you're trying to monitor portions and keep to the calories per serving, you'll know how much to serve.

I truly believe eating healthy is possible without breaking the bank or spending all day cooking. I hope the recipes and tips in this cookbook open up new possibilities in your meal repertoire and help you whip up delicious, healthy meals in a flash. Now, let's get started on cooking five-ingredient dishes. Happy, healthy cooking!

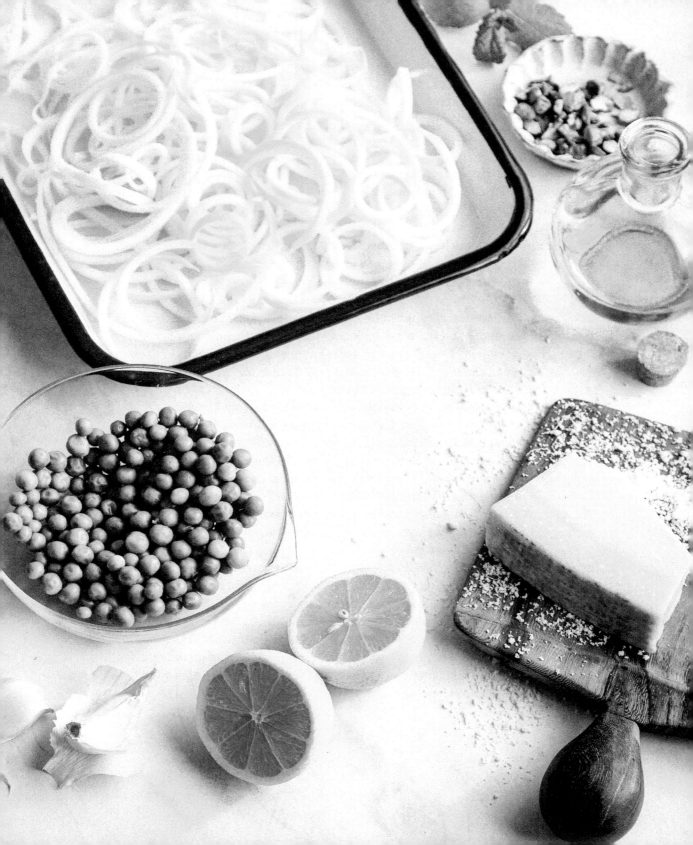

1 Healthy Cooking Made Simple

Y ou don't have to spend the afternoon creating complicated and intricate dishes to enjoy a healthy diet. Believe me, as a single, working mom of three kids, I don't have the time or the desire to spend all day in the kitchen! During my years as a dietitian in private practice, many of my clients were shocked to learn that cooking healthy meals can be really simple. To counter misconceptions about this subject, over the past 10 years, I have shared my simple, healthy recipes on FoodNetwork.com's *Healthy Eats* blog, on MensFitness.com, and in *Muscle & Fitness* magazine. Now I'm happy to share my tips and tricks for cooking healthy with you, right here at your fingertips. In this chapter, we'll explore the basics of healthy cooking and the tools and equipment you will want to have to start cooking clean, healthy, and easy meals right away.

Clean Eating Guidelines

There is no formal definition of *clean eating*; however, it has generally come to mean a diet filled with wholesome foods that are not overly processed and an ingredient list of pronounceable and recognizable ingredients. Many of the foods people eat every day are processed to some degree, and it's not always a bad thing. For example, Greek yogurt is strained to give it a thicker consistency and creamy mouthfeel. Straining also enables the yogurt to have twice the protein and 40 percent less sugar and sodium compared to traditional yogurt. Another example of a food that undergoes some processing is quinoa. This seed (yep, it's a seed!) contains a bitter residue called saponins. Many food companies rinse quinoa before packing it to remove the saponins, making your life in the kitchen a little easier.

Frozen foods can also be clean if you choose the right foods. Food manufacturers freeze fruits and vegetables at their peak of freshness in order to preserve the nutritional value. I love to keep frozen produce stocked in my freezer in case I run low on fresh, or if offerings at the market are limited due to seasonality. When selecting frozen fruits, look for products without added sugar and where the fruit is listed as the only ingredient. Avoid frozen vegetables slathered in creamy sauces, cheese, or butter. If the ingredient list includes anything more than just the vegetable, take a pass on it.

Similarly, canned foods can be part of a clean, healthy diet. A 2016 study published in *Journal of the Academy of Nutrition and Dietetics* found that people who choose canned produce have a better diet, eat more fruits and veggies, and fill up on more key nutrients without going overboard on sodium or gaining weight compared to those who forgo canned produce. This may surprise you. Folks who added canned produce to their diet also took in more fiber, choline, and potassium, and less fat. So which canned foods should you choose? Look for canned vegetables and legumes (such as beans, peas, and lentils) that are low in sodium or have no added sodium. If you do purchase legumes that aren't low in sodium, it's helpful to rinse them before using. A 2011 study published by *Journal of Culinary Science & Technology* found that draining and rinsing canned beans can reduce the sodium content by up to 40 percent. When choosing canned fruits, look for those packed in their own juices or in water. Canned fruits in either heavy or light syrup add unnecessary calories and sugar.

The processed foods worth minimizing are those you can easily whip up yourself, like salsa and salad dressings, and those that are processed to the point where they lose their nutritional value, like potato chips, cookies, and cakes. A clean eating diet focuses on a variety of foods, including whole grains, lean protein, legumes, low- or nonfat dairy, fruits, vegetables, nuts, seeds, and healthy oils, like olive oil.

THE TOP CLEAN, HEALTHY DIETS

Fad diets pop in and out of the headlines. Many tout quick weight loss and appear tempting to follow. Before starting any diet, however, there are a few red flags to look out for. If any diet you are considering raises one or more of these red flags, I encourage you to forget about it, and I'll tell you why:

The diet tells you to avoid one or more food groups. Each food group provides its own variety of important nutrients, and avoiding any of them means missing out on essential elements your body needs.

The diet tells you to buy a whole bunch of supplements. Your medical conditions, overall health, and current medications can interact with supplements. Any diet that tells you to buy hundreds of dollars' worth of supplements without seeking the advice of a physician and registered dietitian can be dangerous.

The diet promises quick weight loss. According to the National Institutes of Health, a safe rate of weight loss is one to two pounds per week. If you lose weight more quickly, make sure you are under the care of a physician. Of course, you also want to keep the weight off, and as the saying goes, "slow and steady wins the race."

The diet doesn't recommend or, even worse, pooh-poohs regular exercise. Regular physical activity is a critical component to any weight-loss plan and to leading an overall healthy lifestyle.

Okay, so which diets are both clean and safe to follow? Here are my top picks:

DASH DIET

Dietary Approaches to Stop Hypertension (DASH) was created by the National Heart, Lung, and Blood Institute to help lower and prevent high blood pressure. The DASH diet promotes foods containing nutrients like potassium, calcium, fiber, and protein that have been shown to help reduce high blood pressure. The plan emphasizes a variety of foods that contain these nutrients, especially fruits, vegetables, whole grains, lean protein, and low-fat dairy. High-fat, high-sodium, and added-sugar foods are discouraged. Although this plan was originally created for those with high blood pressure, the DASH diet has been ranked Best Diet Overall by *U.S. News & World Report* for seven years in a row. This well-balanced diet encourages whole foods and discourages high-calorie and processed foods. The DASH diet also promotes regular exercise and an overall healthy lifestyle, including an emphasis on not smoking.

MEDITERRANEAN DIET

The 2015–2020 Dietary Guidelines for Americans include the Mediterranean diet as a healthy eating pattern. It has also been consistently named one of the Best Diets Overall by *U.S. News & World Report*. This diet touts fruits, vegetables, seafood, lean meat, and plant proteins, like nuts, seeds, and legumes. Conversely, the Mediterranean diet discourages high-fat cuts of meat and processed foods. Exercise is encouraged, as is enjoying the ceremony of mealtime with family and friends.

MIND DIET

The Mediterranean-DASH Intervention for Neurodegenerative Delay (MIND) diet is a cross between the Mediterranean and DASH diets. Developed by researchers at Rush University, this eating plan was created to help lower the risk of Alzheimer's disease by more than one-third. Although the MIND diet was created for cognitive function, it promotes a well-balanced diet filled with wholesome and minimally processed foods. In fact, the diet identifies 10 "brain-healthy food groups" that are high in antioxidants, resveratrol, and healthy fatty acids. These foods include berries, green leafy vegetables, olive oil, nuts, whole grains, fish, and beans. Foods to limit include butter, margarine, pastries, whole-fat cheese, red meat, and fast food. In addition to its cognitive benefits, this plan can also lead to weight loss.

VEGETARIAN DIET

Although following a vegetarian diet has become trendy, it's a diet plan rooted in individual choice. When followed in a healthy manner, it can also lead to weight loss. The 2015–2020 Dietary Guidelines for Americans recognize a vegetarian eating pattern as a healthy diet. Instead of meat, poultry, and seafood, a vegetarian diet promotes soy, legumes, nuts, seeds, whole grains, fruits, and vegetables. Many vegetarians include eggs and dairy; however, you can follow a stricter vegetarian diet that eliminates either or both. If you choose to follow a vegetarian diet, it's important to find alternative protein sources; choose wholesome, less processed foods; and limit added sugars, saturated fat, and high-sodium foods.

CLEAN EATING FOR GOOD HEALTH

If you have a health condition, such as heart disease, diabetes, or obesity, following a clean diet can be particularly helpful. Overly processed foods tend to be higher in added sugar—think cakes and cookies. But there are also hidden sources of added sugar, like barbecue sauce and salad dressing, both of which can be easily made at home so you can control the ingredients. For someone with diabetes, it's all about the sugar, which you're able to better control when you make your own meals, desserts, and condiments. By following a clean diet, you're also minimizing fatty cuts of meat and many prepackaged foods that may be high in calories. Eating foods high in saturated fat, like fatty cuts of meat or fast food, has long been associated with a higher risk of heart disease. Additionally, eating too many calories over a long period of time can lead to obesity.

USING THIS BOOK FOR BETTER HEALTH

If you are trying to eat healthier or lose weight, consider each recipe's nutrition information, including calories, total fat, saturated fat, protein, carbohydrates, fiber, and sodium. You can also keep an eye on each recipe's listed serving size, such as 1 piece, ¼ cup, or 2 tablespoons. This helps guide you in portion control, so you can stick to the amount that's considered a reasonable serving.

Each recipe is also labeled if it meets the criteria for any of the following:

Gluten-Free: These recipes do not contain wheat, rye, or barley. Some ingredients, like oats, do not contain gluten but may be processed in a facility that also processes wheat. Always read the label to check if your food is gluten-free. If it is processed in a facility containing wheat, the label must disclose this information.

Dairy-Free: These recipes do not contain milk or dairy foods, including cheese, ice cream, cottage cheese, and yogurt.

Paleo-Friendly: These recipes do not contain grains, white flour, dairy, legumes, refined sugar, yeast, vinegar, or pickled foods.

Vegan: These recipes do not contain any food derived from an animal, including meat, poultry, seafood, dairy, eggs, and honey.

Vegetarian: These recipes do not contain meat, poultry, or seafood. They may contain eggs and dairy.

Making Healthy Cooking Easy

Although I am a single mother of three with a full-time job, and I also play competitive tennis, I still insist on cooking healthy meals for my family. With limited time to cook, I've come up with quick and easy recipes that can get it done. Healthy cooking *can* be easy and delicious, and in this cookbook, I share my tips and tricks so you can do it, too!

SIMPLE FIVE-INGREDIENT RECIPES

One of the biggest hurdles to healthy cooking is all that shopping. Many recipes call for 10 or more ingredients, which can be overwhelming—a shopping list in itself for just one meal? Ridiculous! Cutting back the ingredients is one simple way to make your life easier. Even better news: Many of your favorite dishes can be made using only five main ingredients! Once you get the hang of these five-ingredient recipes, you can learn to modify them to your liking by adding more ingredients or swapping ingredients. In this cookbook, I present seven items that you should always keep on hand—these don't count toward the five ingredients. These seven items are used in many recipes:

1. Cooking spray

2. Salt

3. Freshly ground black pepper

4. Olive oil

5. Honey

6. Fresh garlic

7. Fresh lemons (fresh because the juice and the zest are frequently used)

Aside from these seven items, each recipe in this book includes no more than five main ingredients. When the five main ingredients appear along with any of these seven items, they are highlighted in the ingredient list.

HEALTHY EATING SHORTCUTS

The following tips can help make healthy eating easier as well as more convenient, enjoyable, and affordable:

Plan, plan, and plan. A little advance planning can go a long way in helping you succeed in your mission. Over the weekend, plan which nights you'll be cooking and select the healthy recipes you want to cook. Also, have all your ingredients ready to go—that is, purchased and prepped—on those nights you choose to cook.

Have a running shopping list. I keep a pad and paper on my kitchen counter so anyone in the house can add a food item we've run out of. Yes, sometimes my kids jot down "CHOCOLATE" or "ICE CREAM" (in all caps), but this list has saved me on more than one occasion. The last thing you want to do is be running to the market on a busy weeknight, and the best way to remember what you have to buy is to write it down.

Meal prep. In addition to advance planning, I love to get some advance cooking done over the weekend. I prepare double batches and freeze half for a busy week when I won't have much time to cook. I also like to prepare sides or soups over the weekend to help minimize the need to cook entire meals throughout the week.

Creatively reuse leftover foods. To help curb food waste, repurpose leftover dishes and ingredients. For example, my Black Bean-Quinoa Burgers (page 91) can be eaten in a bun, but they can also be crumbled over a green salad. Also, you may find that after you prepare a recipe, you have leftover fruits or vegetables, which can then be used to make a salad or a smoothie. Over-ripe fruits that nobody wants to eat anymore, such as avocados or brown bananas, are terrific to peel, freeze, and sneak into a future smoothie.

Schedule meals on your time. Dinner doesn't always have to be at 6 p.m. On school days, dinner is ready and waiting for my kids when they get home from school at 3:30 p.m. Yes, 3:30! I know that when my kids come home from school, they are at their hungriest. Instead of eating mindless snacks until 6 or 7 p.m., they eat a well-balanced meal and then attend their activities or get started on homework. Then at 7 or 8 p.m., when they are hungry again, we enjoy a family snack together. This helps minimize cooking when I'm exhausted and enables me to enjoy time with my kids. Having dinner ready at 3:30 p.m. may not work in your house, but do what works for *you*—not what you *think you need* to be doing. Shift meal and snack times to work within your individual schedule. You'll be patting yourself on the back for your creativity!

The recipes in this cookbook are the perfect way to start practicing these tips and tricks and make healthy cooking easy!

Healthy Cooking Techniques

It's not only the food in the recipe but also how you cook it that makes a difference. Here are some techniques that work well for cooking healthy meals.

Baking: Baking is usually synonymous with desserts and breakfast items, but you can also bake seafood, lean meat, poultry, fruits, and vegetables. Baking doesn't usually require the addition of fat, but it's important to keep an eye on the time to avoid overbaking, which can dry out food. To bake a food, place it in a pan or ovenproof dish, covered or uncovered, for the specified duration of time.

Grilling: This is an excellent way to cook meat, poultry, seafood, vegetables, and fruits. Grilling allows fat to drip off, and it also browns the food, adding flavor.

Poaching: This cooking technique involves submerging food into water or a flavored liquid (like broth) to cook. Fish, eggs, chicken, and some fruits and vegetables can be poached.

Roasting: This technique is used for cooking vegetables as well as larger cuts of meat, poultry, and fish. Roasting brings out flavors in vegetables that can't be duplicated by other methods. When roasting meats, it's recommended to place the meat or poultry on a rack to allow the fat to drip off.

Steaming: This easy method for cooking vegetables, fruits, fish, shellfish, and chicken breasts doesn't require fat. To steam, cover the bottom of a medium pot with water and fit with a steamer basket filled with food. Bring the water to a boil, then reduce to a simmer. Cover the pot and cook until the food is cooked through.

Sautéing: This cooking method uses a small amount of fat to cook food quickly over high heat. When sautéing, use a shallow pan to let the moisture escape and leave room between the food items in the pan.

Stir-frying: Typically used to prepare Asian-style dishes, stir-frying involves cooking small pieces of food over high heat with a small amount of oil. This quick, high-heat method also preserves the crispness, bright color, and nutrients in the food.

HELPFUL KITCHEN EQUIPMENT

To be ready to cook healthy, you'll want to arm yourself with the right supplies. I recommend starting with the "must-have" list. After a few weeks of cooking healthy, easy recipes, you'll have a better idea of what works best for you and can begin exploring the "nice-to-have" supplies.

MUST-HAVES

Baking sheets (or sheet pans): From roasting vegetables to baking meat, poultry, and seafood, rimmed baking sheets will serve as an all-purpose cooking vessel in your healthy kitchen. They're lightweight, inexpensive, and durable. Make sure your kitchen is stocked with at least two.

Blender: You don't need to invest hundreds of dollars on a fancy blender. I bought my first blender on sale by using my Bed Bath & Beyond 20-percent-off coupon! You'll get a lot of use out of your blender making batters, smoothies, sauces, and dips. When cleaning your blender, make sure to take it apart completely so you can properly clean the blender blades.

Sauté pan: A sauté pan has tall sides set at a right angle to the base, which creates a larger bottom surface and protects against splattering. These babies are useful to cook breakfast items, like my Mexican-Style Potato Hash and Eggs (page 22), or a quick dinner, like my Chicken Quesadillas (page 119). I recommend a 12-inch straight-sided sauté pan.

Mixing bowls: A set of three mixing bowls (small, medium, and large) is very useful for mixing, stirring, and folding ingredients together. I still have my first set of stainless-steel mixing bowls that I bought 18 years ago and I use them almost daily!

Cutting boards: Healthy cooking includes lots of fruits and vegetables. To prepare them, you'll have to do some slicing and dicing, which is best done on a cutting board. Your kitchen should be stocked with at least two cutting boards: one for fruits and vegetables and the second for raw meats, poultry, and fish. I prefer plastic cutting boards that can be tossed into the dishwasher.

Measuring cups and spoons: Portion control is key to eating healthy. The ingredient amounts I list in each recipe correspond to the nutrition information. If you overpour oil, for example, it can add hundreds of unnecessary calories to a recipe, since 1 tablespoon of any oil contains 120 calories. The same goes for nuts; if a recipe calls for ¼ cup and you want to adhere to the suggested serving size, measure it out so you don't end up adding hundreds of extra calories to the dish.

NICE-TO-HAVES

Slow cooker: This small appliance is one of the easiest cooking vessels to use and can drastically minimize your time in the kitchen. You don't need a slow cooker with bells and whistles—a simple one goes for around $30.

Good utensils: Once you get in the healthy cooking swing of things, you'll find it's worthwhile to update these kitchen utensil essentials. Good utensils include a spatula, a garlic press, a few wooden spoons (they're usually sold in packs), a lemon juicer, and a ladle. If you use a nonstick pan, opt for a plastic- or silicone-coated spatula to avoid damaging the pan's surface.

Good set of knives: If you've been slicing and dicing fruits and vegetables with a dull knife, you'll be pleasantly surprised how much easier a new, sharp blade makes your food prep. There's no need to spend hundreds of dollars on an elaborate set. I recommend investing in a good chef's knife and a paring knife. A chef's knife is perfect for slicing meat, cutting vegetables, and chopping herbs and nuts. A paring knife is designed for more fine cutting skills, like peeling and slicing kiwi, deseeding peppers, or segmenting orange slices.

Storage containers: Good storage containers are so convenient to have. Look for easily stackable, BPA-free, leakproof containers. Also, make sure they're microwave, freezer, and dishwasher safe, which will allow for easy batch cooking so you can freeze your food and reheat it later. I also recommend adding a few mason jars to your food container collection. Perfect for salads, parfaits, and snacks, they can be easily toted to work.

MEAL PLANNING BASICS

Meal planning can be a lifesaver when you're a busy person trying to eat healthy. This includes planning what you're going to cook, when you're going to shop and cook, and when you're going to eat your healthy meals. Planning keeps you organized and makes healthier eating easier. Meal planning also saves money because you'll be working from an exact shopping list of foods you need, which will minimize your impulse purchases, runs to fast-food joints, and expensive takeout orders.

Here are step-by-step instructions for creating and executing a weekly meal plan and shopping list:

1. Choose one day during the weekend when you will be preparing meals.

2. Select five to seven healthy recipes. I like to choose one breakfast, two main dishes, two sides, and one snack. The number of recipes you choose to cook depends on how much time you have.

3. Using each recipe, create a shopping list according to the flow of the super-market. Check your pantry, refrigerator, and freezer to make sure you don't already have an ingredient on hand. I usually divide my shopping list by fruits, vegetables, dairy, pantry items, and frozen goods.

4. Go food shopping the day before you will cook. I find it takes at least 90 minutes to go shopping and put the food away at home.

5. Start cooking your dishes. I always start the slow cooker recipe (if I have one) first, and then move on to the most time-consuming dish. While that dish is cooking, I prep vegetables or the more simple dishes.

6. Once each dish is complete, store it in single-serve portions in the refrigera-tor or freezer, depending on how soon you would like to eat or serve it. I divide salads into single-serve portions so I can easily grab them on my way to work.

7. Keep a folder with recipes you love, or put sticky notes in the cookbook (for example, *The kids loved this one!*) so you're reminded to make them again.

Pantry Essentials

A well-stocked pantry can make healthy cooking a breeze. That doesn't mean you need to overstock your pantry—then your goodies will get lost in the crowd. Rather, keep it organized and clean, and keep track of the use-by dates so you can use products with the earliest expiration dates first. A well-stocked pantry can also minimize your time at the supermarket and can curb how much you spend if you keep it organized. On more than one occasion, when my pantry got a little messy, I ended up buying a duplicate product because I didn't see that it was already in my pantry.

As a reminder, the following are seven essential items that will be required to prepare the recipes in this book. These items do not count toward the five main ingredients used in the recipes, and they will be used repeatedly throughout many of the recipes. The first five items are nonperishable, and the last two can be stored for several weeks.

1. Cooking spray

2. Salt

3. Freshly ground black pepper

4. Olive oil

5. Honey

6. Fresh garlic

7. Fresh lemons

SMART SHOPPING TIPS

Stick to the list. When food shopping, always make a shopping list and commit to sticking to it. I suggest a self-imposed rule of no more than two food items not on the shopping list as last-minute indulgent purchases. If you tend to be sucked in by impulse buys during the shopping experience, you may find shopping from home a better option. It's hard to be impulsive when the items aren't right in front of you, tempting you!

Prep for savings. Before heading to the market, check the online app, circulars, and coupons for the foods you need. Many manufacturers offer coupons directly on their websites.

Use a smaller cart. It can be tempting to fill the cart to the brim. Using a smaller cart can prevent unnecessary overshopping.

Shop manager's specials. Shop the butcher's counter for manager's specials. The meats sold on special are safe to eat and offer a nice discount. You usually do need to cook them right away, however.

Look around. The most expensive items tend to be placed at eye level. You may find better buys at the top and bottom of the shelves.

Dig deep. Although the outer perimeter of the store has the fresh produce, dairy, butcher counter, and other wholesome foods, don't count out the inside aisles, which stock many healthy foods, like nuts, healthy oils, canned beans and lentils, and frozen produce.

Shop smartly in bulk. Some foods are smart to purchase in bulk, like a large bag of quinoa—*if* you eat it regularly. However, if you purchase large portions of nuts thinking you'll save money in the long run, they may actually spoil before you get a chance to eat them all. This depends on your household usage. Some foods I like to buy in bulk include olive oil, cooking spray, salt, black pepper, and honey.

Compare labels. If you're debating between two or three brands, take a few minutes to compare the labels to see which has more of the good stuff, like fiber, calcium, and vitamin D, and less of the not-so-good stuff, like saturated fat, sodium, and added sugar.

Buy seasonal produce. If you're looking to save money on fruits and vegetables, check the chart on page 14 for what's in season. Whether you buy at your supermarket or local farmers' market, fruits and vegetables tend to be cheaper when in season.

Don't fall in the "free of" trap. Many foods tout the fact that they are free of gluten, dairy, sugar, eggs, and so on. I often question what *is* in these products rather than what isn't. Unless you have a specific food allergy, don't fall for the "free of" laundry list on labels. Instead, think about the nutrients you need to keep you healthy and if this food contains what you need.

Source inexpensive nutrition. Expensive isn't always healthier. Some foods touted as superfoods, like acai and chia seeds, carry a high price tag, but the truth is, you can get the same nutrients in more readily accessible foods that are much cheaper.

Seasonal Produce Guide

The following chart can help you discern when fresh, local ingredients are in season. Purchasing fruits and vegetables in season can help you save money, so keep your eyes peeled for these foods throughout the year. Although many foods are included on this chart, you may find a few delicious surprises pop up at your local market that are not listed here, depending on where you live and shop—so take advantage of them, too! Please note that seasonality of fruits and vegetables varies throughout the country.

SPRING	SUMMER	FALL	WINTER
MAR–MAY	JUN–AUG	SEP–NOV	DEC–FEB
Apricots	Apricots	Acorn squash	Brussels sprouts
Artichokes	Beets	Belgian endive	Grapefruit
Asparagus	Bell peppers	Broccoli	Kale
Broccoli	Blackberries	Butternut squash	Leeks
Chives	Blueberries	Cabbage	Oranges
Collard greens	Cherries	Cauliflower	Parsnips
Fava beans	Corn	Cranberries	Squash (many winter varieties)
Fennel	Eggplant	Garlic	Tangerines
Green beans	Figs	Pears	Turnips
Peas	French beans	Pumpkin	
Radicchio	Garlic	Rutabagas	
Rhubarb	Jalapeño peppers	Sweet potatoes	
Snow peas	Lima beans	Swiss chard	
Sorrel	Peaches		
Strawberries	Peas		
Swiss chard	Plums		
Watercress	Shallots		
	Tomatillos		
	Tomatoes		
	Watermelon		
	Zucchini		

About the Recipes

The recipes in this cookbook contain up to five main ingredients, and may also use any of the seven items you should always keep on hand (see page 12). In addition, at least half of the recipes in this cookbook can be prepared in a single vessel, in 30 minutes or less, in a slow cooker, or are freezer friendly. These recipes will be tagged with any of these labels:

One Pot/One Pan: These recipes can be made in a single pot, bowl, pan, or piece of equipment (like a smoothie in a blender).

30-Minute: These recipes can be prepared, cooked, and served in 30 minutes or less.

Slow Cooker: These recipes can be made in a slow cooker.

Freezer-Friendly: These recipes can be made ahead of time and frozen for easy heating later. These recipes will include storage and reheating instructions.

Each recipe will list the total servings or yield and the nutrition information for one serving. The nutrition information provided includes the calories, total fat, saturated fat, protein, carbohydrates, fiber, and sodium. Every recipe will also have a Toby's Tip, which will give you a healthy cooking hack, tip, or trick to enhance the flavor, prep an ingredient a different way, store the dish, or substitute other interesting ingredients. I always have a great time creating Toby's Tips and hope you have fun using them!

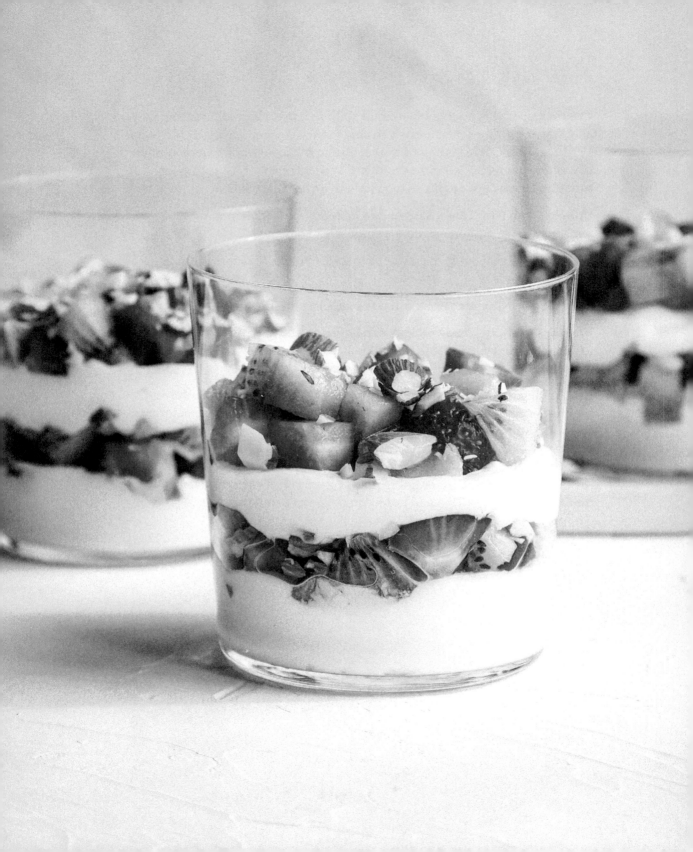

2 Smoothies and Breakfasts

Blueberry-Spinach Smoothie

GLUTEN-FREE | VEGETARIAN

I'm always looking for delicious ways to add vegetables into my breakfast. Years ago, a friend suggested adding vegetables to my morning smoothie. I was hesitant at first, worried that the smoothie wouldn't taste fruity or sweet, like I prefer. However, once I discovered this combo of blueberries, apple juice, and spinach, there was no turning back.

SERVES 1

ONE POT/ONE PAN
30-MINUTE

Prep time: 5 minutes

1 cup frozen blueberries

2 cups spinach, washed and patted dry

½ cup nonfat plain Greek yogurt

½ cup 100% apple juice

1 teaspoon honey

In a blender, add the blueberries, spinach, yogurt, apple juice, and honey, and blend until smooth. Pour into a tall glass and serve.

TOBY'S TIP: When purchasing frozen fruit, make sure it has no added sugar by reading through the ingredient list or looking for "No added sugar" on the label.

Serving size: 14 fluid ounces
Per serving: Calories: 232; Total fat: 1g; Saturated fat: 0g; Protein: 14g; Carbohydrates: 45g; Fiber: 6g; Sodium: 99mg

Grape-Melon Smoothie

GLUTEN-FREE | DAIRY-FREE | VEGETARIAN

The fruits I use in this smoothie tend to be the ones that I always have a little extra of in my refrigerator. One morning I decided to toss some melon and grapes in my blender, and voilà, this pretty, green-hued smoothie was born. The tart lime balances the flavor of the sweet melon. If you have super ripe, sweet melon, you can leave the honey out.

SERVES 1

ONE POT/ONE PAN
30-MINUTE

Prep time: 10 minutes

1 cup diced honeydew

1 cup diced cantaloupe

1 cup green seedless grapes

¼ cup 100% orange juice

Juice of 1 lime

1 teaspoon honey

In a blender, add the honeydew, cantaloupe, grapes, orange juice, lime juice, and honey, and blend until smooth. Pour into a tall glass and serve.

TOBY'S TIP: Thoroughly rinse and scrub the outside of melons before slicing. The rind contains grooves that trap dirt and potentially dangerous bacteria. These bacteria can get onto your melon when you slice through it. Use a stiff-bristle brush to get all the dirt off.

Serving size: 16 fluid ounces
Per serving: Calories: 242; Total fat: 1g; Saturated fat: 0g; Protein: 3g; Carbohydrates: 61g; Fiber: 4g; Sodium: 45mg

Tropical Protein Smoothie

Cottage cheese is one of the most underappreciated foods, even though it contributes both texture and nutrition to a dish. One-half cup of low-fat cottage cheese provides 97 calories, 3 grams of fat, 13 grams of protein, and 4 grams of carbs. Many folks don't realize how protein-packed it is. When blended, its texture becomes smooth and creamy, making it a perfect ingredient to add to a smoothie.

SERVES 1

**ONE POT/ONE PAN
30-MINUTE**

Prep time: 5 minutes

¾ cup diced frozen pineapple

¾ cup fresh baby kale, rinsed and patted dry

¾ cup diced fresh or frozen mango

½ cup low-fat cottage cheese

½ cup skim milk or light coconut milk

1 teaspoon honey

In a blender, add the pineapple, kale, mango, cottage cheese, milk, and honey, and blend until smooth. Pour into a tall glass and serve.

TOBY'S TIP: Save money and reduce food waste by freezing leftover pineapple, mango, and other fruits—don't let those brown bananas go to waste, either! Cut into 1- to 1½-inch cubes, place on a tray in a single layer, and freeze. Once frozen, transfer to a resealable plastic bag in the freezer for up to 4 months.

Serving size: 16 fluid ounces
Per serving: Calories: 349; Total fat: 4g; Saturated fat: 1g; Protein: 21g; Carbohydrates: 60g; Fiber: 7g; Sodium: 445mg

Cherry-Banana Smoothie

GLUTEN-FREE | VEGETARIAN

In my constant search for flavor combinations using easy-to-find foods, I fell in love with bananas and cherries. I always have bananas on hand in my kitchen for my pre-tennis snack, and when they're not in season, I keep a bag of frozen pitted cherries in my freezer. Cherries provide a healthy dose of vitamins A and C and contain two inflammation-fighting antioxidants, anthocyanin and quercetin.

SERVES 1

**ONE POT/ONE PAN
30-MINUTE**

Prep time: 5 minutes

1 medium banana

½ cup frozen pitted
sweet cherries

½ cup nonfat plain
Greek yogurt

½ cup nonfat milk
or almond milk

½ teaspoon vanilla extract
or ground nutmeg

In a blender, add the banana, cherries, yogurt, milk, and vanilla or ground nutmeg, and blend until smooth. Pour into a tall glass and serve.

TOBY'S TIP: Swap the banana for 1 cup frozen berries for a delicious cherry-berry smoothie.

Serving size: 14 fluid ounces
Per serving: Calories: 255; Total fat: 0g; Saturated fat: 0g; Protein: 17g; Carbohydrates: 49g; Fiber: 5g; Sodium: 98mg

Mexican-Style Potato Hash and Eggs

GLUTEN-FREE | VEGETARIAN

I love the combination of Mexican flavors at breakfast. With a limit of five ingredients, it was tough to choose which of those flavors to use in this dish. I opted for avocado and cilantro to add some healthy fat and the refreshing flavor of fresh herbs. This well-balanced dish is a perfect way to start your morning for a reasonable 320 calories per serving.

SERVES 6

ONE POT/ONE PAN

Prep time: 20 minutes

Cook time: 25 minutes

3 large russet potatoes

2 tablespoons olive oil

½ teaspoon salt

¼ teaspoon freshly ground black pepper

6 large eggs

6 tablespoons shredded pepper Jack cheese

1 avocado, pitted, peeled, and cubed

6 tablespoons chopped fresh cilantro

1. Peel and grate the potatoes, and drain the excess liquid.

2. Preheat the broiler.

3. In a large, oven-safe skillet over medium-high heat, heat the olive oil. When the oil is shimmering, add the grated potatoes. Cook the potatoes, stirring occasionally, until slightly browned and cooked through, about 10 minutes. Add the salt and pepper, and toss to combine.

4. Using a wooden spoon, create 6 evenly spaced wells in a circular pattern in the potato hash. Crack 1 egg into a wineglass. Gently pour the egg into a well. Repeat with the remaining eggs. Reduce heat to medium-low, cover the skillet, and cook until the eggs are cooked through, about 12 minutes.

5. Uncover the skillet, and sprinkle each egg with 1 tablespoon of cheese. Place the uncovered skillet in the broiler for 2 minutes, until the cheese has melted and is slightly browned. Remove from the broiler.

6. On each of 6 plates, spoon 1 egg with one-sixth of the hash on a plate. Top each with 1 tablespoon of avocado and 1 tablespoon of chopped cilantro and serve.

TOBY'S TIP: Dress up your Mexican-Style Potato Hash and Eggs by adding salsa or sriracha, black beans, and a dollop of reduced-fat sour cream.

Serving size: 1 egg plus ⅙ of the hash

Per serving: Calories: 320; Total fat: 17g; Saturated fat: 4g; Protein: 12g; Carbohydrates: 33g; Fiber: 7g; Sodium: 345mg

Egg in a Hole

In college, I was thrilled when a sweet boy I liked invited me over for a home-cooked breakfast. When we sat down to eat, he served what appeared to be a slice of toasted bread. I kept wondering, Why is this guy staring at me, waiting to eat this slice of toasted bread? He then told me to cut the bread with the fork and knife he provided. I cautiously sliced it open and lo and behold, I found the egg inside. That was the first time I ever ate an Egg in a Hole, and I have been making this dish regularly ever since.

SERVES 4

ONE POT/ONE PAN
30-MINUTE

Prep time: 10 minutes

Cook time: 10 minutes

4 slices 100% whole-wheat bread

2 teaspoons unsalted butter, at room temperature

Cooking spray

4 large eggs

1 (¾-ounce) slice provolone cheese

1 tomato, cut crosswise into 4 slices

¼ teaspoon salt

⅛ teaspoon freshly ground black pepper

1. Using a cookie cutter or the top of a round glass, cut a hole in the center of each slice of bread. Reserve the centers of the bread for another use.

2. Spread ½ teaspoon of butter on each of the slices of bread.

3. Coat a nonstick skillet with cooking spray and heat over medium-high heat. When the cooking spray is shimmering, place the bread (buttered-side up) in the skillet. Crack 1 egg into a wineglass. Gently pour the egg into the center hole of 1 slice of bread. Repeat with the 3 remaining eggs and bread. Cook until the eggs are set, about 3 minutes, and carefully flip over each piece.

4. Gently place 1 slice of cheese and 1 slice of tomato onto egg, and continue cooking an additional 3 minutes, until the eggs are cooked through and the cheese has slightly melted. Sprinkle the top of each tomato slice with salt and pepper. Serve immediately.

TOBY'S TIP: For an extra kick, top your Egg in a Hole with my Mediterranean Chopped Salad (page 41). Melt the cheese as directed (without the tomato), and place the Egg in a Hole on a plate. Top with ½ cup of the chopped salad.

Serving size: 1 egg in a hole
Per serving: Calories: 228; Total fat: 14g; Saturated fat: 7g; Protein: 14g; Carbohydrates: 13g; Fiber: 2g; Sodium: 333mg

Broccoli-Cheddar Egg Muffins

GLUTEN-FREE | VEGETARIAN

It's no surprise that broccoli is good for you. But you may not know that eggs contain an important nutrient called choline, which is needed for a healthy liver, athletic performance, brain function, and proper neurological development. According to the Choline Council and recent National Health and Nutrition Examination Survey data, about 90 percent of Americans don't get enough choline. Foods that include eggs, like these delicious egg muffins, are one of the best sources.

SERVES 12

FREEZER-FRIENDLY

Prep time: 15 minutes

Cook time: 30 minutes

Equipment: Steamer basket

Cooking spray

2 cups broccoli florets

12 large eggs

½ cup skim milk or almond milk

3 scallions, chopped

½ teaspoon salt

¼ teaspoon freshly ground black pepper

¾ cup shredded low-fat Cheddar cheese

1. Preheat the oven to 350°F. Spray 12 muffin liners with cooking spray or place a liner in each cup of a 12-muffin tin.

2. Fill a medium pot with about an inch of water. Fit a steamer basket into the pot, and add the broccoli florets. Cover and heat over medium-high heat about 5 minutes, until the broccoli is crisp. Transfer the broccoli to a cutting board and allow to cool for 5 minutes, then chop the florets.

3. In a large bowl, whisk together the eggs, milk, scallions, salt, and pepper. Add the chopped broccoli, and toss to combine.

4. Spoon ⅓ cup of egg mixture into each of the prepared muffin liners, and top each with 1 tablespoon of shredded cheese.

5. Bake until the tops are golden brown, about 25 minutes. Let the muffins cool for 10 minutes before removing them from the tin. Serve while still warm.

6. To freeze, place the egg muffins in a single row in a freezer-safe container in the freezer for up to 2 months. To defrost, refrigerate overnight. Reheat in a 350°F oven for 5 to 10 minutes. Alternatively, reheat egg muffins in the microwave on high for 45 to 60 seconds and allow them to cool for 2 minutes before eating.

TOBY'S TIP: Reduce food waste by using whatever leftover veggies you have on hand, like mushrooms, peppers, cauliflower, or spinach.

Serving size: 1 muffin

Per serving: Calories: 100; Total fat: 6g; Saturated fat: 2g; Protein: 9g; Carbohydrates: 2g; Fiber: 0g; Sodium: 229mg

Flourless Peanut Butter–Apple Muffins

GLUTEN-FREE | DAIRY-FREE | VEGETARIAN

It used to be that every time I ate a muffin, I felt hungry right after. Rather than give up my beloved muffins, I wanted to find a way to increase my satiety by adding protein and fat, which take longer to digest. The answer to my dilemma: nut butter. I now use it as the main ingredient in my muffins and complement the flavor with fruit, like apples, pears, strawberries, and blueberries.

SERVES 12

30-MINUTE
FREEZER-FRIENDLY

Prep time: 10 minutes

Cook time: 15 minutes

Cooking spray

⅔ cup natural creamy peanut butter

2 large eggs

½ cup plus 2 tablespoons packed brown sugar

1 teaspoon baking powder

1 apple, cored and diced

1. Preheat the oven to 350°F. Coat a 12-cup muffin tin with cooking spray.

2. In a medium bowl, whisk together the peanut butter, eggs, brown sugar, and baking powder until smooth.

3. Gently fold the apple into the batter until evenly distributed.

4. Scoop ¼ cup of batter into each prepared muffin cup, filling each cup halfway. Tap the bottom of the muffin tin on the counter 2 or 3 times to release any air bubbles.

5. Bake for about 15 minutes, until the muffins are golden brown on top and a toothpick inserted in the center comes out clean.

6. Remove from the oven and allow to cool for 5 minutes. Transfer the muffins to a wire rack and let cool for another 10 minutes.

TOBY'S TIP: Mix and match 1 cup of your favorite fruit with peanut butter or almond butter to create the flavor combo you love. For a boost of flavor, add 1 teaspoon each of vanilla extract and ground cinnamon.

Serving size: 1 muffin
Per serving: Calories: 148; Total fat: 8g; Saturated fat: 2g; Protein: 5g; Carbohydrates: 16g; Fiber: 1g; Sodium: 122mg

Banana–Chocolate Chip Waffles

I steer clear of waffle mixes, as I like to make my own. However, most DIY waffle batter recipes contain a lot more than five ingredients! Using nut butter, eggs, and banana, this recipe makes a deliciously easy batter that's filled with enough protein and healthy fat to help keep you satisfied throughout any busy morning.

SERVES 8

FREEZER-FRIENDLY

Prep time: 10 minutes

Cook time: 25 minutes

Equipment: Waffle iron

Cooking spray

2 medium ripe
bananas, mashed

2 large eggs

½ cup smooth almond butter

½ teaspoon baking soda

¼ cup semisweet
chocolate chips

1. Preheat a standard waffle iron and coat with cooking spray.

2. In a blender, add the mashed bananas, eggs, almond butter, and baking soda, and blend until smooth. Transfer the batter to a medium bowl, and gently fold in the chocolate chips until evenly distributed.

3. Pour 1 cup of batter onto the waffle iron, and cook for 3 minutes on each side. Transfer the cooked waffle to a plate, and repeat with the remaining batter to make a total of 4 waffles. To freeze, store waffles in a freezer-safe container in the freezer for up to 3 months. To defrost, refrigerate overnight. Reheat in the microwave on high for 30 to 45 seconds and allow waffles to cool for 2 minutes before eating. Alternatively, reheat waffles in a toaster oven.

TOBY'S TIP: Top your waffle with nonfat plain Greek yogurt and fresh fruit or chopped nuts.

Serving size: ½ waffle
Per serving: Calories: 353; Total fat: 24g; Saturated fat: 4g; Protein: 12g; Carbohydrates: 29g; Fiber: 5g; Sodium: 139mg

Strawberry-Kiwi Yogurt Parfaits

I love to liven up my yogurt by layering it in a visually appealing parfait. First, I choose my yogurt base (usually nonfat plain or vanilla), then select my fruit combo (like strawberry-banana, strawberry-kiwi, or apple-pear), and top it with some crunch (granola, nuts, or whole-grain cereal). The result is always a mouthwatering, well-balanced, and very pretty breakfast.

SERVES 4

30-MINUTE

Prep time: 15 minutes

1 cup (about 8 large) strawberries, hulled and diced

2 kiwis, peeled and diced

¼ cup freshly squeezed or 100% orange juice

1 (32-ounce) container nonfat vanilla Greek yogurt

½ cup almonds, chopped

1. In a small bowl, place the strawberries and kiwis. Add the orange juice, and toss to evenly coat.

2. In each of 4 parfait glasses, layer ½ cup yogurt and top with 2 tablespoons of the fruit mixture, followed by 1 tablespoon of chopped almonds. Repeat for a second layer.

3. Serve, or cover and refrigerate for up to 3 days.

TOBY'S TIP: For a grab-and-go breakfast, assemble these parfaits in mason jars with lids.

Serving size: 1 parfait
Per serving: Calories: 314; Total fat: 9g; Saturated fat: 1g; Protein: 23g; Carbohydrates: 40g; Fiber: 4g; Sodium: 78mg

Apple-Pecan Sorghum Porridge

GLUTEN-FREE | VEGETARIAN

Let me introduce you to this ancient hot grain. Thought to have originated in Africa, sorghum can grow in areas with little or no water. This feature has made sorghum one of the most important cereal crops in the world. One-quarter cup of uncooked sorghum provides 158 calories, 5 grams protein, 35 grams carbohydrates, and 3 grams fiber. It's also a good source of iron, providing about 12 percent of the recommended daily amount.

SERVES 4

**ONE POT/ONE PAN
FREEZER-FRIENDLY**

Prep time: 10 minutes

Cook time: 1 hour

4 cups skim milk

1 cup dry sorghum

¼ teaspoon salt

2 tablespoons
100% maple syrup

½ cup raw pecans, chopped

1 medium apple,
cored and diced

1. In a medium saucepan over medium heat, bring the milk to a gentle boil, stirring occasionally.

2. Add the sorghum and salt, and cover. Bring to a boil, stirring occasionally. Reduce heat to low and continue cooking, covered, until the sorghum is tender and fluffy, about 50 minutes.

3. Add the maple syrup and stir to combine. Fold in the pecans and apple until evenly distributed. Serve warm.

4. To freeze, store porridge in a freezer-safe container in the freezer for up to 2 months. To defrost, refrigerate overnight. Reheat individual portions in the microwave on high for 1 to 2 minutes. To reheat on the stovetop, heat the entire batch of porridge in a saucepan over medium heat for about 5 to 8 minutes, until heated through.

TOBY'S TIP: To cut cooking time, use pearly sorghum, which takes only 25 minutes to cook. You can also swap out the sorghum for quinoa or barley, and cook per package instructions.

Serving size: 1 cup*
Per serving: Calories: 381; Total fat: 11g; Saturated fat: 1g; Protein: 15g; Carbohydrates: 63g; Fiber: 5g; Sodium: 255mg
*Please note: The nutrition information for sorghum is only available for dry sorghum, not cooked sorghum.

Pumpkin Pie Oatmeal

GLUTEN-FREE | VEGETARIAN

In the fall, I love baking pumpkin pie with my girls, but I always get stuck with leftover pumpkin purée. Instead of tossing it, I add the leftover purée to a variety of dishes, including my morning oatmeal.

SERVES 4

**ONE POT/ONE PAN
30-MINUTE**

Prep time: 5 minutes

Cook time: 10 minutes

2 cups gluten-free
quick-cooking rolled oats

4 cups skim milk or
almond milk

1 cup pumpkin purée

1 teaspoon pumpkin
pie spice

3 tablespoons
100% maple syrup

1. In a medium pot over high heat, combine the oats and milk. Bring the mixture to a boil, stirring occasionally. Lower heat to medium and cook, stirring occasionally, until the oats begin to soften and the liquid thickens, about 7 minutes. Remove from heat.

2. Stir in the pumpkin purée, pumpkin pie spice, and maple syrup until evenly distributed. Serve warm.

TOBY'S TIP: Be sure to choose pumpkin purée as opposed to pumpkin pie mix, which is drowning in added sugar. Pumpkin purée will list pumpkin as the only ingredient.

Serving size: 1¼ cups
Per serving: Calories: 294; Total fat: 4g; Saturated fat: 1g; Protein: 14g; Carbohydrates: 54g; Fiber: 7g; Sodium: 107mg

Slow Cooker Pear-Cinnamon Oatmeal

GLUTEN-FREE | VEGETARIAN

I prepare breakfast for my kids every morning, no exceptions. But some nights I end up working very late and need those extra 15 minutes to sleep in. That's when my slow cooker comes to the rescue. I toss in some steel-cut oats, a liquid, spices, and fruit, and let the slow cooker do its job. Steel-cut oats are heartier than the quick-cooking oats and hold up well in the slow cooker. By morning, my kids can serve themselves a healthy, delicious breakfast, and I can hit the snooze button a few more times.

SERVES 6

SLOW COOKER

Prep time: 10 minutes

Cook time: 7 hours

Cooking spray

2 cups gluten-free steel-cut oats

2 cups water

2 cups nonfat milk or almond milk

¾ teaspoon cinnamon

2 medium pears, cored and diced

1 tablespoon honey

1. Coat the inside of the slow cooker with cooking spray.

2. Evenly spread the oats in the bottom of the slow cooker.

3. In a medium bowl, whisk together the water, milk, and cinnamon. Add the pears, and toss to combine. Pour the mixture over the oats.

4. Set the slow cooker on low, and cook for 7 hours.

5. Once the oatmeal is cooked, stir in the honey. If the oatmeal is too thick, loosen it with additional milk.

TOBY'S TIP: Check the label on the oats for the phrase *gluten-free*. Some oats are processed in facilities that also process gluten-filled products, which can cause a reaction for those with a gluten allergy.

Serving size: About 1 cup

Per serving: Calories: 273; Total fat: 3g; Saturated fat: 1g; Protein: 10g; Carbohydrates: 52g; Fiber: 7g; Sodium: 37mg

Simple Blueberry-Banana Pancakes

DAIRY-FREE | VEGETARIAN

Pancakes are my kids' favorite, but some mornings I have limited time to whip them up. That's when these five-ingredient pancakes come in handy. You can swap the blueberries for chocolate chips, sliced strawberries or peaches, or chopped almonds or pecans.

SERVES 4

30-MINUTE
FREEZER-FRIENDLY

Prep time: 10 minutes

Cook time: 10 minutes

4 medium ripe bananas, mashed

4 large eggs, lightly beaten

½ cup whole-wheat pastry flour

½ teaspoon ground cinnamon

1 cup fresh or thawed frozen blueberries

Cooking spray

1. In a medium bowl, mix together the mashed bananas, beaten eggs, flour, and cinnamon until evenly combined. Gently fold in the blueberries.

2. Coat a griddle or large skillet with cooking spray and place over medium heat. Once hot, ladle ¼ cup of batter at a time onto the griddle or skillet, leaving room between the pancakes. Cook until the top is bubbly and the edges are set, about 2 minutes.

3. Flip the pancakes and cook until golden brown and crisp along the edges, about 2 minutes. Remove and keep warm by covering with aluminum foil or placing in the oven at the lowest setting until ready to serve. Repeat with the remaining batter.

4. To freeze, store in a freezer-safe container in the freezer for up to 3 months. To defrost, refrigerate overnight. Reheat in the microwave on high for 30 to 45 seconds and allow the pancakes to cool for 2 minutes before eating. Alternatively, reheat pancakes in a toaster oven.

TOBY'S TIP: If you like your pancakes to have a very smooth mouthfeel, as opposed to a little chunkiness with the mashed bananas, blend the batter before adding the blueberries.

Serving size: 3 pancakes
Per serving: Calories: 253; Total fat: 6g; Saturated fat: 2g; Protein: 9g; Carbohydrates: 44g; Fiber: 6g; Sodium: 73mg

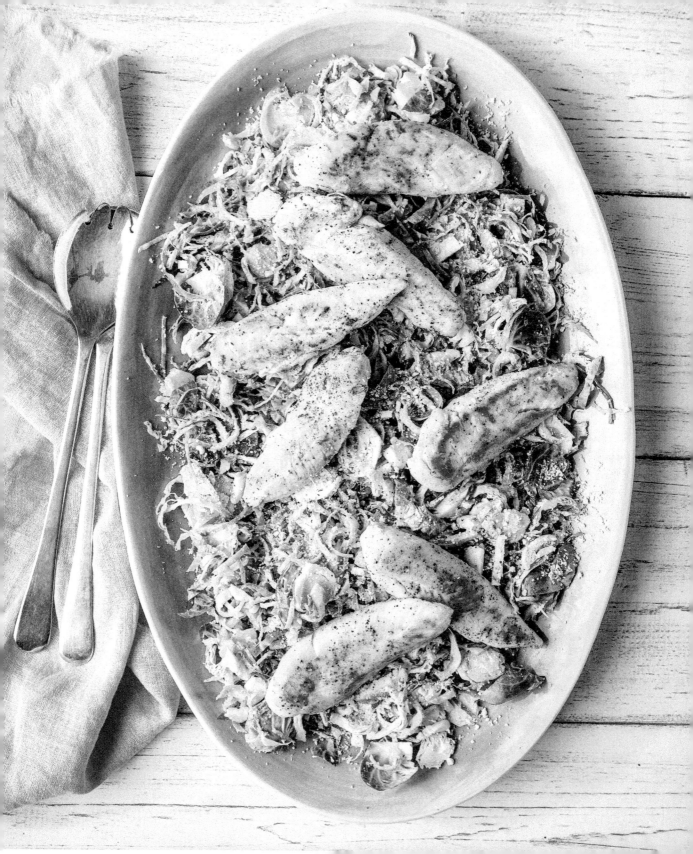

3

Hearty Soups and Salads

Silky Tomato Soup

I am the oldest of five children, so when my mom needed to feed her brood, she, too, turned to easy and tasty meals. One of my favorites was tomato soup, which she usually paired with grilled cheese. When I created this tomato soup, I kept my mom in mind— she, like many parents, had a full-time job but always cooked for us.

SERVES 4

FREEZER-FRIENDLY

Prep time: 15 minutes

Cook time: 45 minutes

1 tablespoon olive oil

1 onion, chopped

2 garlic cloves, minced

2 (28-ounce) cans crushed tomatoes

2 cups low-sodium vegetable broth or chicken broth

¼ teaspoon freshly ground black pepper

¼ cup fresh basil leaves, cut into ribbons

1. In a large saucepan over medium heat, heat the olive oil. When the oil is shimmering, add the onion and garlic and cook for about 3 minutes, until the onion is translucent and the garlic is fragrant. Add the tomatoes, broth, and pepper, and bring to a boil. Reduce heat and simmer, covered, until the flavors come together, about 40 minutes.

2. Remove from heat. Add the basil leaves. Pour the soup into a blender or use an immersion blender to carefully blend the ingredients until smooth. Return the soup to the saucepan to keep warm if serving immediately.

3. To freeze, allow the soup to cool to room temperature for up to 2 hours, then store in a resealable container in the freezer for up to 2 months. To defrost, refrigerate overnight. To reheat on the stovetop, bring to a boil over medium-high heat, then lower heat to medium-low and simmer for 10 minutes until heated through. Alternatively, reheat single-serve portions in the microwave on high for 2 to 3 minutes.

TOBY'S TIP: Up your protein and fiber intake by adding some cooked whole grains like quinoa, sorghum, or brown rice.

Serving size: About 2 cups
Per serving: Calories: 176; Total fat: 5g; Saturated fat: 1g; Protein: 8g; Carbohydrates: 32g; Fiber: 8g; Sodium: 880mg

Creamy Carrot and Chickpea Soup

Chickpeas get lots of attention for their starring role in hummus, but there's much more you can do with them. One of my cooking hacks is to add chickpeas to a soup for a healthy dose of protein, fiber, folate, iron, and zinc. You can add them whole, but chickpeas also blend beautifully into soups, creating a creamy texture and mouthfeel.

SERVES 4

ONE POT/ONE PAN
FREEZER-FRIENDLY

Prep time: 10 minutes

Cook time: 25 minutes

2 tablespoons olive oil

8 carrots, cut into
½-inch-thick rounds

1 onion, finely chopped

3 garlic cloves, minced

1 tablespoon grated
fresh ginger

1 (15-ounce) can
low-sodium chickpeas

5 cups low-sodium chicken
broth or vegetable broth

¼ teaspoon salt

⅛ teaspoon freshly
ground black pepper

1. In a medium saucepan over medium heat, warm the olive oil. Add the carrots and onion, and sauté for 5 minutes until both are softened.

2. Add the garlic and ginger, and cook for 1 minute, stirring frequently.

3. Add the chickpeas with their liquid, broth, salt, and pepper, and bring the mixture to a boil.

4. Reduce heat and simmer for 15 minutes.

5. Using an immersion blender or traditional blender, carefully purée the soup until smooth.

6. Serve warm or freeze for later. If freezing, allow the soup to cool to room temperature for up to 2 hours, then store in a resealable container in the freezer for up to 2 months. To defrost, refrigerate overnight. To reheat on the stovetop, bring to a boil over medium-high heat, then lower heat to medium-low and simmer for 10 minutes until heated through. Alternatively, reheat single-serve portions in the microwave on high for 2 to 3 minutes.

TOBY'S TIP: Dress up this soup with a dollop of reduced-fat Greek yogurt and a sprinkle of smoked paprika.

Serving size: 1¾ cups

Per serving: Calories: 203; Total fat: 8g; Saturated fat: 1g; Protein: 10g; Carbohydrates: 31g; Fiber: 9g; Sodium: 763mg

Slow Cooker Corn and Sweet Potato Chowder

GLUTEN-FREE | DAIRY-FREE | VEGAN | VEGETARIAN

I was always afraid of using a slow cooker, and started using one only a few years ago. I still am shocked at how easy it is! You toss in all the ingredients, cover, and set. After a few hours, you get delicious dishes—in this case, a killer chowder. I don't know how I ever survived without my slow cooker, but I will never go without it again.

SERVES 4

SLOW COOKER
FREEZER-FRIENDLY

Prep time: 20 minutes
Cook time: 2 hours on high or 3½ hours on low

1 tablespoon olive oil

1 onion, finely diced

2 garlic cloves, minced

2 sweet potatoes, peeled and diced

1 pound frozen corn

4 cups low-sodium vegetable broth or chicken broth

½ teaspoon salt

⅛ teaspoon freshly ground black pepper

1. In a medium sauté pan or skillet over medium heat, heat the olive oil. When the oil is shimmering, add the onion and sauté for 3 minutes.

2. Add the garlic and sauté for 1 minute, stirring frequently.

3. Transfer the onion and garlic to a slow cooker. Top with the sweet potatoes, corn, broth, salt, and pepper.

4. Cover and cook for 2 hours on high or 3½ hours on low.

5. Using an immersion blender or traditional blender, carefully purée the chowder until mostly smooth, leaving some chunks of vegetables.

6. Serve warm or freeze for later. To freeze, allow the soup to cool to room temperature for up to 2 hours, then store in a resealable container in the freezer for up to 2 months. To defrost, refrigerate overnight. To reheat on the stovetop, bring to a boil over medium-high heat, then lower heat to medium-low and simmer for 10 minutes until heated through. Alternatively, reheat single-serve portions in the microwave on high for 2 to 3 minutes.

TOBY'S TIP: For added flavor and color, top this chowder with 2 tablespoons of Easy Pesto Sauce (page 185).

Serving size: 1¾ cups
Per serving: Calories: 232; Total fat: 5g; Saturated fat: 1g; Protein: 9g; Carbohydrates: 40g; Fiber: 5g; Sodium: 475mg

Protein-Packed Parsnip and Pea Soup

GLUTEN-FREE | DAIRY-FREE | VEGAN | VEGETARIAN

When I was a girl, my mother served up pea soup regularly, and I was not a fan. As a stubborn youngster, I would sit at the table leaving the soup untouched until I had permission to leave the table. As an adult, I've learned to punch up pea soup to my liking. Parsnips add a sweet flavor to the peas, and I also add tofu to boost the protein. The result is *the best* pea soup I have ever tried—hey, even chefs can give kudos to themselves once in a while!

SERVES 4

FREEZER-FRIENDLY

Prep time: 10 minutes

Cook time: 30 minutes

2 tablespoons olive oil

1 large onion, diced

4 parsnips, peeled and diced

8 ounces silken tofu, cubed

2 (10-ounce) packages (about 4 cups) frozen peas

3 cups low-sodium vegetable broth

½ teaspoon salt

¼ teaspoon freshly ground black pepper

1. In a medium saucepan over medium heat, heat the olive oil. When the oil is shimmering, add the onion and parsnips, and cook for about 10 minutes, until the parsnips soften and the onion is translucent.

2. Add the tofu and cook until it softens, about 2 minutes.

3. Add the frozen peas and cover with the vegetable broth. Bring to a boil, reduce heat, and simmer, covered, for about 15 minutes, until the peas soften. Add the salt and pepper and stir to combine.

4. Transfer the soup to a blender or use an immersion blender, and carefully blend until almost smooth, leaving chunks of vegetables.

5. Serve warm or freeze for later. To freeze, cool to room temperature up to 2 hours, then transfer to a resealable container and store in the freezer for up to 2 months. To defrost, refrigerate overnight. To reheat on the stovetop, bring to a boil over medium-high heat, then lower heat to medium-low and simmer for 10 minutes until heated through. Alternatively, reheat single-serve portions in the microwave on high for 2 to 3 minutes.

TOBY'S TIP: For a nonvegetarian option, substitute chicken broth for the vegetable broth.

Serving size: 2 cups
Per serving: Calories: 294; Total fat: 9g; Saturated fat: 1g; Protein: 12g; Carbohydrates: 42g; Fiber: 12g; Sodium: 566mg

Cauliflower-Turmeric Soup

GLUTEN-FREE | DAIRY-FREE | VEGAN | VEGETARIAN

Turmeric is a relative to ginger and is a main ingredient in curry powder. One table-spoon of this yellow-orange spice has 24 calories and 1 gram each of fat, fiber, and protein, plus 15 percent of the daily recommended amount of iron. This bad boy also contains the potent antioxidant curcumin, shown to help fight inflammation.

SERVES 4

FREEZER-FRIENDLY

Prep time: 15 minutes

Cook time: 30 minutes

1 tablespoon olive oil

1 large onion, chopped

3 garlic cloves, chopped

1 large russet potato, peeled and diced

1 cauliflower head, chopped into florets

4 cups low-sodium vegetable broth

1 teaspoon turmeric powder

½ teaspoon salt

¼ teaspoon freshly ground black pepper

1. In a large pot over medium heat, heat the olive oil. When the oil is shimmering, add the onion and garlic, and cook for about 5 minutes, until the onion is translucent and the garlic is fragrant. Add the potato and cauliflower, and sauté for about 10 minutes, until softened.

2. Add the broth, turmeric, salt, and pepper, and bring to a boil. Reduce heat and simmer, covered, for about 15 minutes, until the vegetables soften and the flavors combine.

3. Use an immersion blender or pour the soup into a blender, and carefully blend until smooth.

4. Serve warm or freeze for later. To freeze, cool to room temperature up to 2 hours, then transfer to a resealable container and store in the freezer for up to 2 months. To defrost, refrigerate overnight. To reheat on the stovetop, bring to a boil over medium-high heat, then lower heat to medium-low and simmer for 10 minutes until heated through. Alternatively, reheat single-serve portions in the microwave on high for 2 to 3 minutes.

TOBY'S TIP: After refrigeration or freezing, soups may become a little thicker. You can thin them out by adding water, low-sodium broth, or skim milk as needed.

Serving size: 1¾ cups
Per serving: Calories: 165; Total fat: 4g; Saturated fat: 1g; Protein: 6g; Carbohydrates: 27g; Fiber: 6g; Sodium: 905mg

Leftover Chicken Soup

GLUTEN-FREE | DAIRY-FREE | PALEO-FRIENDLY

Every Friday night, my mom would prepare chicken soup made from scratch, stock and all. Sometimes I do have a few hours to kill and prepare a DIY stock, but for the most part I use a low-sodium chicken broth and fill it with leftover chicken and a mirepoix: a combo of onions, celery, and carrots. This soup has become a go-to, especially during a busy workweek.

SERVES 4

ONE POT/ONE PAN

Prep time: 10 minutes

Cook time: 25 minutes

1 tablespoon olive oil

1 onion, chopped

2 garlic cloves, minced

1 medium carrot, chopped

1 celery stalk, chopped

8 ounces cubed leftover chicken, rotisserie chicken (without the skin), or Easy Sautéed Chicken Breast (page 118)

6 cups low-sodium chicken broth

¼ teaspoon freshly ground black pepper

1. In a large pot over medium heat, heat the olive oil. When the oil is shimmering, add the onion, garlic, carrot, and celery, and cook for 4 minutes, until the onion is translucent.

2. Add the chicken and stir to combine. Add the broth and pepper, and mix together. Increase heat to high and bring to a boil. Reduce heat, cover, and simmer for about 20 minutes, until the flavors combine.

TOBY'S TIP: Dress up your chicken soup by adding frozen peas or fresh leeks, parsnips, and turnips.

Serving size: 1⅔ cups

Per serving: Calories: 311; Total fat: 25g; Saturated fat: 6g; Protein: 18g; Carbohydrates: 5g; Fiber: 1g; Sodium: 438mg

Deconstructed Guacamole Salad

GLUTEN-FREE | DAIRY-FREE | PALEO-FRIENDLY | VEGAN | VEGETARIAN

Writing this cookbook with a limited number of ingredients really had me thinking. For classic dishes like guac, which ingredients stay and which go? It's exactly what I had to do when creating this Deconstructed Guacamole Salad, and the results are holy wow!

SERVES 4

**ONE POT/ONE PAN
30-MINUTE**

Prep time: 15 minutes

Zest and juice of 2 limes

½ teaspoon salt

⅛ teaspoon freshly ground black pepper

3 ripe avocados, pitted, peeled, and diced

1½ cups grape tomatoes, halved

¼ red onion, diced

¼ cup chopped fresh cilantro

1. In a medium bowl, whisk the lime zest and juice, salt, and pepper.

2. Add the diced avocado and gently toss with the lime mixture.

3. Add the tomatoes, onion, and cilantro, then gently toss again.

4. Serve immediately.

TOBY'S TIP: To speed the ripening of an avocado, place it in a brown paper bag with an apple or banana for 2 to 3 days.

Serving size: About 1 cup
Per serving: Calories: 257; Total fat: 22g; Saturated fat: 3g; Protein: 4g; Carbohydrates: 17g; Fiber: 11g; Sodium: 309mg

Mediterranean Chopped Salad

GLUTEN-FREE | DAIRY-FREE | PALEO-FRIENDLY | VEGAN | VEGETARIAN

My mom is Israeli, and every summer when I was growing up, she rented an apartment in Israel for our family to live in for two months, usually in Ashkelon, where she is from. We would live among the locals and spend time with my mother's extended family, attend camp, and learn the language. Every day she made us a chopped salad with cucumbers, tomatoes, and peppers. In each of my cookbooks, you'll find a spinoff of my chopped salad that I still eat regularly. This version has chopped olives, which are usually on an Israeli table at every meal, including breakfast.

SERVES 4

ONE POT/ONE PAN
30-MINUTE

Prep time: 15 minutes

⅔ cup chopped hothouse cucumber

2 plum tomatoes, chopped

1 red bell pepper, chopped

½ red onion, chopped

⅓ cup pitted Kalamata olives, halved lengthwise

1 tablespoon olive oil

Juice of 1 lemon

¼ teaspoon salt

⅛ teaspoon freshly ground black pepper

1. In a medium bowl, add the cucumber, tomatoes, bell pepper, onion, and olives. Toss to combine.

2. Add the olive oil, lemon juice, salt, and pepper, and toss evenly to coat the vegetables.

TOBY'S TIP: Enjoy this salad as a side to the Green Shakshuka (page 90), Braised Cod over Tomatoes (page 107), or Slow Cooker Rosemary-Lemon Chicken with Potatoes and Carrots (page 130).

Serving size: About 1 cup
Per serving: Calories: 77; Total fat: 6g; Saturated fat: 0g; Protein: 2g; Carbohydrates: 7g; Fiber: 2g; Sodium: 252mg

Kale and Green Cabbage Salad

GLUTEN-FREE | DAIRY-FREE | VEGAN | VEGETARIAN

Recently I was at dinner with friends when one of them whispered to me that she doesn't like kale because it's too bitter and a tougher green. Oh, the madness! Calmly, I assured her she isn't the first to dislike kale, but knowing how to prepare it can help. Kale becomes much softer after it comes into contact with an acidic ingredient, like a dressing. After making a kale salad, pour on the dressing and let it sit in the refrigerator for at least 15 minutes—out comes a whole new side of this leafy green.

SERVES 6

ONE POT/ONE PAN
30-MINUTE

Prep time: 20 minutes

8 cups chopped kale or baby kale

2 cups shredded green cabbage

½ cup Raspberry Vinaigrette (page 175)

1 medium apple, cored and thinly sliced

½ cup dried cranberries

1. In a large bowl, toss together the kale and cabbage.

2. Add the Raspberry Vinaigrette and toss to evenly coat. Cover and refrigerate for at least 15 minutes.

3. Remove the bowl from the refrigerator. Add the sliced apple and cranberries, and toss to combine.

TOBY'S TIP: Make this salad your own with any of the following swaps: spinach for the kale, red cabbage for the green, pear for the apple, or dried tart cherries or raisins for the cranberries.

Serving size: 2 cups
Per serving: Calories: 222; Total fat: 15g; Saturated fat: 2g; Protein: 4g; Carbohydrates: 22g; Fiber: 5g; Sodium: 141mg

Hearts of Palm, Tomato, and Black Bean Salad

Hearts of palm isn't an ingredient I usually have in my pantry, so I tend to order it as part of my salad when I visit my local deli. But after I found myself spending 11 dollars on these salads numerous times a week, I finally realized that I could easily make the salad at home for only a few dollars.

SERVES 4

30-MINUTE

Prep time: 15 minutes

Cook time: 0 minutes

8 cups shredded romaine lettuce

1 (14-ounce) can hearts of palm, drained and rinsed

1 cup grape tomatoes, halved lengthwise

¾ cup canned low-sodium black beans, drained and rinsed

½ cup Lighter Green Goddess Dressing (page 179)

1. In a large bowl, combine the shredded lettuce, hearts of palm, tomatoes, and black beans.

2. Drizzle with the dressing and toss evenly to coat.

TOBY'S TIP: To tote this salad to work, don't dress the salad. Instead, place 2 tablespoons of the dressing into each of 4 glass mason jars. Fill each jar with about 3 cups of salad. Refrigerate for up to 3 days, and shake well before eating.

Serving size: About 3 cups salad, plus 2 tablespoons dressing
Per serving: Calories: 116; Total Fat: 2g; Saturated Fat: 0g; Protein: 10g; Carbohydrates:19g; Fiber: 8g; Sodium: 479mg

Watermelon Salad with Feta and Mint

GLUTEN-FREE | VEGETARIAN

This refreshing salad brings together the delicious flavors of bounteous summer watermelon, tomatoes, and mint. I'll whip it up for an outdoor barbecue, where many of my guests are pleasantly surprised by the savory use of watermelon.

SERVES 8 AS A SIDE OR 4 AS A MAIN

Prep time: 15 minutes

Cook time: 25 minutes

1 cup pearl barley

3 cups water

6 cups cubed watermelon

1 cup grape tomatoes, quartered

3 tablespoons olive oil

Zest and juice of 1 lemon

1 garlic clove, minced

3 tablespoons chopped fresh mint

¼ teaspoon salt

⅛ teaspoon freshly ground black pepper

1 cup reduced-fat crumbled feta

1. In a medium pot over high heat, bring the barley and water to a boil. Reduce heat to low, cover, and simmer for about 25 minutes, until the water is absorbed and the barley is soft and fluffy. Drain off any excess water and allow the barley to slightly cool for 10 minutes.

2. In a large bowl, toss together the watermelon and tomatoes.

3. In a small bowl, whisk together the olive oil, lemon zest and juice, garlic, mint, salt, and pepper. Pour the dressing over the barley, and toss to combine.

4. Gently fold the barley into the watermelon and tomatoes.

5. Sprinkle the feta on top and serve.

TOBY'S TIP: With its combination of whole grains, dairy, vegetable, and fruit, this salad can double as a side dish for fish or chicken, or be enjoyed as a main dish on its own.

Serving size: 1 cup as a side, 2 cups as a main

Per serving (as a side): Calories: 210; Total fat: 8g; Saturated fat: 2g; Protein: 7g; Carbohydrates: 30g; Fiber: 5g; Sodium: 324mg

Per serving (as a main): Calories: 419; Total fat: 16g; Saturated fat: 5g; Protein: 14g; Carbohydrates: 60g; Fiber: 11g; Sodium: 648mg

Strawberry Caprese Salad

GLUTEN-FREE | VEGETARIAN

There's nothing sweeter than picking a fresh strawberry from a field and taking a juicy bite. It's truly nature's candy. I'm lucky enough to have visited many strawberry fields throughout California, where about 90 percent of the strawberries in the United States are grown.

SERVES 4

ONE POT/ONE PAN
30-MINUTE

Prep time: 15 minutes

3 cups (about 24) strawberries, hulled and halved

8 ounces mozzarella cheese, diced

¼ cup fresh basil leaves, cut into ribbons

¼ cup Balsamic Vinaigrette (page 174)

1. In a medium bowl, toss together the strawberries and mozzarella cheese. Sprinkle with the basil.

2. Drizzle the Balsamic Vinaigrette over the salad, and toss to combine.

TOBY'S TIP: For a traditional caprese salad, swap the strawberries for tomatoes.

Serving size: 1 cup
Per serving: Calories: 299; Total fat: 23g; Saturated fat: 9g; Protein: 13g; Carbohydrates: 10g; Fiber: 2g; Sodium: 439mg

White Bean and Arugula Salad

GLUTEN-FREE | DAIRY-FREE | VEGETARIAN

Arugula is a member of the cabbage family and is brimming with antioxidant vitamins A and C. It also contains the antioxidant lutein, which helps maintain healthy eyes, skin, and hair. The other ingredients deliver their own benefits, including protein, fiber, vitamins B_{12} and K, copper, and some additional vitamins A and C to boot.

SERVES 4

ONE POT/ONE PAN
30-MINUTE

Prep time: 15 minutes

5 cups arugula, rinsed and patted dry

1 (15-ounce) can low-sodium cannellini beans, drained and rinsed

¼ red onion, thinly sliced

1 cup grape tomatoes, halved lengthwise

½ cup Orange Dressing (page 176)

1. In a large bowl, combine the arugula, beans, onion, and tomatoes.

2. Drizzle with the dressing and toss to evenly coat.

TOBY'S TIP: Arugula is sold in different forms: in bunches with the roots attached, loose in bins, or packaged in ready-to-serve containers. Store fresh arugula wrapped tightly in a plastic bag in the refrigerator for up to 2 days. Ready-to-serve containers of arugula should be stored in the refrigerator immediately after returning from the market.

Serving size: 1½ cups
Per serving: Calories: 311; Total fat: 19g; Saturated fat: 3g; Protein: 9g; Carbohydrates: 29g; Fiber: 6g; Sodium: 163mg

Green Salad with Poached Salmon

GLUTEN-FREE

Omega-3 fats found in fatty fish, like salmon, have been shown to help support brain and eye health. DHA (docosahexaenoic acid), one of the most common omega-3s found in fatty fish, makes up a significant percentage of fat in the brain and is important for brain development. As for the eyes, the body's highest concentration of DHA is found in the retina, which makes this omega-3 essential for eye health.

SERVES 4

30-MINUTE

Prep time: 5 minutes

Cook time: 25 minutes

2 bay leaves

1 teaspoon peppercorns

1 pound salmon

8 cups mixed greens

½ cup Goat Cheese Dressing (page 182)

1. In a medium saucepan or high-sided skillet over high heat, bring 8 cups of water to a boil. Add the bay leaves and peppercorns. Add the salmon, making sure it's completely covered by the water, and bring the water back to a boil.

2. Cook the salmon for 1 minute, then turn off heat and cover. Let the salmon poach for 20 minutes. With a slotted spoon, carefully remove the fish from the pan and let it cool.

3. Divide the greens between 4 plates. Drizzle 2 tablespoons of dressing over each salad.

4. Cut the salmon into 4 equal pieces, and place one piece on top of each salad.

TOBY'S TIP: To speed up prep time, poach the salmon in advance and keep in the refrigerator for up to 3 days.

Serving size: 2 cups salad plus 1 piece salmon

Per serving: Calories: 313; Total fat: 11g; Saturated fat: 3g; Protein: 34g; Carbohydrates: 14g; Fiber: 8g; Sodium: 180mg

Brussels Sprout Caesar Salad with Chicken

Who said playing with food can't be fun? Brussels sprouts have always been a vegetable that I loved roasted, until I realized you can shred them, which I love even more! Once you add the dressing, either enjoy the salad right away or refrigerate for a few hours, which will soften the Brussels sprouts.

SERVES 4

30-MINUTE

Prep time: 20 minutes

Cook time: 10 minutes

1 pound chicken tenders

½ teaspoon salt

⅛ teaspoon freshly ground black pepper

Cooking spray

1 pound Brussels sprouts, shredded (shred yourself or purchase preshredded)

½ cup Lighter Caesar Dressing (page 178)

½ cup grated Parmesan cheese

1. Season both sides of the chicken with the salt and pepper.

2. Heat a large skillet coated with cooking spray over medium-high heat. When the cooking spray is shimmering, add the chicken tenders and cook for 5 minutes on one side, then flip and cook for an additional 5 minutes.

3. In a large bowl, add the Brussels sprouts and drizzle with the dressing. Toss to evenly coat. Sprinkle with the Parmesan cheese and top with the cooked chicken.

TOBY'S TIP: Swap the sautéed chicken for poached salmon (see page 47) or a hardboiled egg, or just enjoy sans the protein as a side.

Serving size: 1 cup salad plus 3 ounces chicken
Per serving: Calories: 320; Total fat: 18g; Saturated fat: 4g; Protein: 32g; Carbohydrates: 12g; Fiber: 4g; Sodium: 773mg

Steak Salad

When I go out to eat, I tend to order salads. However, I shy away from steak salads, as they are significantly more expensive compared to other choices on the menu. Instead of completely resisting my craving for a good steak salad, I make my own using a lean cut of beef tenderloin, which I can grill on my stovetop grill pan any time of the year.

SERVES 4

30-MINUTE

Prep time: 15 minutes

Cook time: 15 minutes

Cooking spray

12 ounces beef tenderloin

1 tablespoon olive oil

¼ teaspoon salt

¼ teaspoon freshly ground black pepper

8 cups baby spinach, washed and patted dry

½ hothouse cucumber, halved lengthwise and cut into ½-inch half moons

2 plum tomatoes, halved lengthwise and cut into ½-inch half moons

½ cup Dijon Dressing (page 177)

1. Heat a grill or a grill pan coated with cooking spray.

2. Brush the beef tenderloin with olive oil, and sprinkle with salt and pepper.

3. Grill for 10 to 15 minutes, turning occasionally, until browned on all sides with an internal temperature of 145°F.

4. Remove the beef from the grill and allow to cool for 10 minutes, then thinly slice.

5. In 4 individual salad bowls, arrange the baby spinach, cucumber, and tomatoes, and top each salad with about 3 ounces of sliced beef. Drizzle each with 2 tablespoons of dressing and serve.

TOBY'S TIP: Have extra veggies in the refrigerator? Don't let them go to waste. Toss shredded carrots, bell peppers, celery, radishes, broccoli, or any other vegetable you've got on top.

Serving size: About 2½ cups salad plus 3 ounces beef and 2 tablespoons dressing
Per serving: Calories: 353; Total fat: 27g; Saturated Fat: 5g; Protein: 21g; Carbohydrates: 12g; Fiber: 3g; Sodium: 400mg

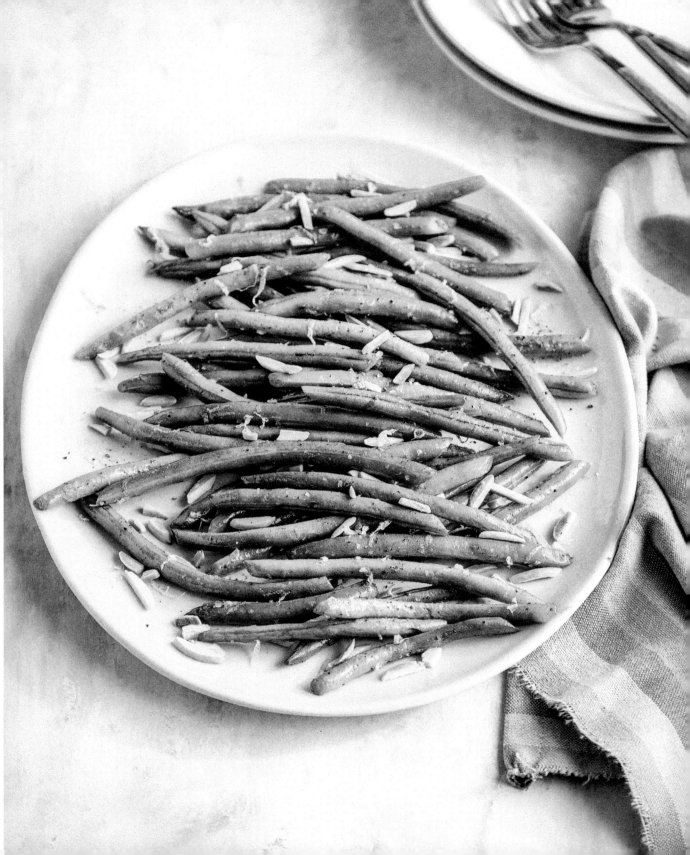

4 Easy Appetizers and Sides

Kickin' Avocado Dip

GLUTEN-FREE | VEGETARIAN

The creamy texture of avocado makes for a mouth-pleasing dip. Paired with the healthy fat and boatload of good-for-you nutrients that avocado provides, it's a win for your taste buds and your body.

MAKES 1 CUP

ONE POT/ONE PAN
30-MINUTE

Prep time: 10 minutes

2 ripe avocados, halved and pitted

¼ cup nonfat plain Greek yogurt

½ jalapeño pepper, seeded

¼ cup roughly chopped fresh cilantro

Juice of 1 lime

½ teaspoon salt

⅛ teaspoon freshly ground black pepper

1. Scoop out the avocado flesh and place it in a blender.

2. Add the yogurt, jalapeño, cilantro, lime juice, salt, and pepper, and blend until smooth.

TOBY'S TIP: After handling jalapeños, make sure to wash your hands thoroughly and avoid touching your eyes, which can get irritated from the jalapeño.

Serving size: ¼ cup
Per serving: Calories: 170; Total fat: 15g; Saturated fat: 2g; Protein: 3g; Carbohydrates: 10g; Fiber: 7g; Sodium: 307mg

Stuffed Jalapeños

GLUTEN-FREE | VEGETARIAN

I made a batch of these spicy pieces of deliciousness, and my boyfriend ended up eating the whole batch. That night, his tummy didn't like all that spiciness, but surprisingly he woke up the next morning asking for more.

SERVES 6

30-MINUTE

Prep time: 10 minutes

Cook time: 10 minutes

Cooking spray

½ cup whipped cream cheese

⅔ cup shredded reduced-fat sharp Cheddar cheese

2 scallions, white and green parts finely chopped

¼ teaspoon salt

⅛ teaspoon freshly ground black pepper

6 large jalapeño peppers, seeded and ribs removed

1. Preheat the oven to 450°F. Coat a baking sheet with cooking spray.

2. In a medium bowl, mix together the cream cheese, Cheddar cheese, scallions, salt, and pepper.

3. Spoon 1 tablespoon of the cream cheese mixture into each jalapeño half, and place on the prepared baking sheet, leaving 1 inch between jalapeño halves.

4. Bake until jalapeños are slightly browned, about 10 minutes.

TOBY'S TIP: Add 1 or 2 slices of chopped cooked bacon to the cream cheese mixture.

Serving size: 2 pieces
Per serving: Calories: 81; Total fat: 6g; Saturated fat: 4g; Protein: 4g; Carbohydrates: 2g; Fiber: 1g; Sodium: 250mg

Cucumber "Bruschetta" with Tomatoes and Olives

If tomato-olive bruschetta is on the menu, you know I'm ordering it! Sometimes, however, I want the delicious flavor without the carbs (which I save for dessert!). I started making my own version at home, swapping out the crusty bread for vegetable coins, like cucumbers or carrots. This helps me shave a few calories off my appetizer, and it's a charming way to add even more veggies to my diet.

SERVES 5

30-MINUTE

Prep time: 20 minutes

1 hothouse cucumber

2 plum tomatoes, diced

2 tablespoons Kalamata olives, chopped

1 tablespoon chopped fresh basil

1 tablespoon olive oil

1 teaspoon balsamic vinegar

1 garlic clove, minced

¼ teaspoon salt

⅛ teaspoon freshly ground black pepper

1. Slice the cucumber on an angle about ½ inch thick for a total of 20 slices.

2. In a medium bowl, combine the tomatoes, olives, and basil.

3. In a small bowl, whisk together the olive oil, vinegar, garlic, salt, and pepper.

4. Pour the olive oil mixture over the tomato mixture, and toss to evenly coat.

5. Spoon 1 teaspoon of tomato mixture over a slice of cucumber and place on a serving platter. Repeat with the remaining cucumber slices.

TOBY'S TIP: To make the tomato mixture even more flavorful, make up to 24 hours in advance and store covered in the refrigerator until ready to use.

Serving size: 4 pieces
Per serving: Calories: 48; Total fat: 3g; Saturated fat: 0g; Protein: 1g; Carbohydrates: 5g; Fiber: 1g; Sodium: 147mg

Lemony Green Beans with Almonds

GLUTEN-FREE | DAIRY-FREE | PALEO-FRIENDLY | VEGAN | VEGETARIAN

Every Thanksgiving, my very large family gathers at my parents' house to celebrate the big feast. Because the guest list has grown to more than 20, my mom requests that everyone bring a dish. I tend to get assigned the vegetable dish, and green beans are one of my go-to choices.

SERVES 4

30-MINUTE

Prep time: 15 minutes

Cook time: 10 minutes

Equipment: Steamer basket

1 pound green beans

½ cup slivered almonds

1 tablespoon olive oil

Zest and juice 1 lemon

¼ teaspoon salt

⅛ teaspoon freshly ground black pepper

1. Fill a medium pot with about an inch of water. Fit a steamer basket into the pot, and bring to a boil over high heat. Add the green beans, cover, and reduce heat to medium. Cook for 5 minutes, until the green beans are tender. Remove from heat and cool for at least 5 minutes.

2. Heat a large skillet over medium-low heat. Add the almonds and cook until slightly browned, about 3 minutes. Remove almonds from the skillet and set aside.

3. Add the green beans, olive oil, lemon zest and juice, salt, and pepper, and stir to combine. Cook for 2 minutes, until the juice is evaporated and the mixture is heated through. Sprinkle the toasted almonds on top.

TOBY'S TIP: Look for loose green beans, which will allow you to pick the freshest ones. Choose slender beans that are brightly colored, firm, and free of brown specks and blemishes. Store green beans tightly wrapped in a plastic bag in the refrigerator for up to 5 days.

Serving size: 1 cup

Per serving: Calories: 145; Total fat: 10g; Saturated fat: 1g; Protein: 5g; Carbohydrates: 11g; Fiber: 5g; Sodium: 154mg

Spicy Roasted Broccoli with Garlic

GLUTEN-FREE | DAIRY-FREE | PALEO-FRIENDLY | VEGAN | VEGETARIAN

Broccoli, a member of the cabbage family, is packed with antioxidant vitamins A and C and a touch of almost every other vitamin and mineral. Broccoli also contains certain plant compounds, like indoles and isothiocyanates, shown to help fight cancer.

SERVES 4

30-MINUTE

Prep time: 15 minutes

Cook time: 15 minutes

1 pound broccoli, cut into bite-size florets

4 garlic cloves, thinly sliced

¼ cup olive oil

¼ teaspoon salt

⅛ teaspoon freshly ground black pepper

⅛ teaspoon red pepper flakes

1. Preheat the oven to 450°F. Line a baking sheet with parchment paper or aluminum foil.

2. In a large bowl, add the broccoli florets and garlic. Toss to combine.

3. In a small bowl, whisk together the olive oil, salt, pepper, and red pepper flakes. Pour the olive oil mixture over the broccoli, tossing to evenly coat.

4. Spread the broccoli on the prepared baking sheet in a single layer. Bake for about 12 minutes, until the broccoli is slightly browned.

TOBY'S TIP: When purchasing, look for broccoli heads with bright green florets and firm stalks. The cut ends of the stalks should appear moist and fresh. Avoid broccoli with brown stems or yellowing florets. Store fresh broccoli, unwashed, in an open plastic bag in the refrigerator for up to 10 days.

Serving size: About ¾ cup
Per serving: Calories: 163; Total fat: 14g; Saturated fat: 2g; Protein: 3g; Carbohydrates: 9g; Fiber: 3g; Sodium: 186mg

Sheet Pan Asparagus with Tomatoes and Pine Nuts

Roasted veggies deliver a whole different experience than their raw counterparts. The red and green hues of these vegetables mixed together with the crunch of pine nuts make this a beautiful, simple, and delicious side dish.

SERVES 4

30-MINUTE

Prep time: 15 minutes

Cook time: 15 minutes

2 tablespoons olive oil

2 garlic cloves, minced

¼ teaspoon salt

⅛ teaspoon freshly ground black pepper

1 pound asparagus, trimmed

1½ cups cherry tomatoes

¼ cup pine nuts

¼ cup grated Parmesan cheese

1. Preheat the oven to 400°F.

2. In a small bowl, whisk together the olive oil, garlic, salt, and pepper.

3. In a large bowl, add the asparagus, tomatoes, and pine nuts. Toss to combine. Drizzle the olive oil mixture over the asparagus, and toss to evenly coat.

4. Spread the asparagus mixture in a single layer on a baking sheet. Roast until the asparagus and tomatoes are tender, about 15 minutes.

5. Transfer to a large serving bowl and sprinkle with the Parmesan cheese.

TOBY'S TIP: To ensure the asparagus cooks evenly, choose asparagus spears that are relatively even in diameter.

Serving size: 4 or 5 asparagus spears plus ¼ cup tomato mixture

Per serving: Calories: 179; Total fat: 15g; Saturated fat: 2g; Protein: 7g; Carbohydrates: 8g; Fiber: 3g; Sodium: 249mg

Sautéed Spinach with Shallots

GLUTEN-FREE | DAIRY-FREE | PALEO-FRIENDLY | VEGAN | VEGETARIAN

As a working mother of three busy kids, I don't have much time to get a healthy meal on the table. Quick and easy recipes, like this one, come in handy. It's all about the simple add-ins, like shallots, that give this side dish a flavorful punch.

SERVES 4

ONE POT/ONE PAN
30-MINUTE

Prep time: 5 minutes

Cook time: 15 minutes

1 tablespoon olive oil

1 shallot, chopped

1 (10-ounce) package frozen spinach, thawed and drained

¼ teaspoon salt

⅛ teaspoon freshly ground black pepper

1. In a medium skillet over medium heat, heat the olive oil. Add the shallot and cook until fragrant, about 2 minutes.

2. Add the spinach, breaking up any remaining frozen pieces with a wooden spoon, and cook until heated through, about 10 minutes.

3. Sprinkle with the salt and pepper, and toss to combine.

TOBY'S TIP: Use 1 pound of fresh spinach instead of a 10-ounce package to yield the same amount.

Serving size: ¼ cup
Per serving: Calories: 54; Total fat: 3g; Saturated fat: 0g; Protein: 2g; Carbohydrates: 4g; Fiber: 3g; Sodium: 257mg

Roasted Potato Medley with Sriracha

GLUTEN-FREE | DAIRY-FREE | PALEO-FRIENDLY | VEGAN | VEGETARIAN

I'm always trying to find ways to use up extra foods I have lying around. I always seem to have a few potatoes, so I slice and roast them. The results are one of the easiest sides to whip up, and one of my family's favorites.

SERVES 4

30-MINUTE

Prep time: 10 minutes

Cook time: 20 minutes

1 large russet potato, peeled

1 large sweet potato, peeled

3 medium red potatoes, cut into ½-inch-thick rounds

2 tablespoons olive oil

1 teaspoon sriracha

½ teaspoon salt

¼ teaspoon freshly ground black pepper

1. Preheat the oven to 425°F. Line a baking sheet with parchment paper or aluminum foil.

2. Halve the russet and sweet potatoes lengthwise, then cut into ½-inch-thick pieces.

3. Place all the potatoes into a large bowl.

4. In a small bowl, whisk the olive oil, sriracha, salt, and pepper.

5. Drizzle the olive oil mixture over the potatoes, tossing to evenly coat.

6. Spread the potato slices in a single layer on the prepared baking sheet. Roast for about 20 minutes, until potatoes are slightly golden.

TOBY'S TIP: Variety is key here, so use whatever potatoes you have lying around, including purple, Yukon, and gold potatoes.

Serving size: 1 cup
Per serving: Calories: 265; Total fat: 7g; Saturated fat: 1g; Protein: 5g; Carbohydrates: 47g; Fiber: 6g; Sodium: 381mg

Sautéed Polenta with Salsa

GLUTEN-FREE | DAIRY-FREE | VEGAN | VEGETARIAN

When I was a bachelorette living in New York City, I needed to find simple, easy meals that I could finish on my own. That's when I became obsessed with precooked polenta. It was easy to cook up and top with a variety of delicious flavors, so I never got bored.

SERVES 6

30-MINUTE

Prep time: 10 minutes

Cook time: 10 minutes

1 (1.1-pound) package precooked polenta, cut into ½-inch-thick rounds

2 tablespoons olive oil

¼ teaspoon salt

⅛ teaspoon freshly ground black pepper

Cooking spray

¾ cup Simple Salsa (page 189)

1. Brush both sides of the polenta rounds with the olive oil, and sprinkle with the salt and pepper.

2. Coat a large sauté pan or a griddle with cooking spray and heat over medium heat. When the cooking spray is shimmering, add the polenta rounds and cook on one side until slightly browned, about 4 minutes, then flip and cook the other side for an additional 3 to 4 minutes.

3. Serve the polenta rounds with spoonfuls of Simple Salsa on top.

TOBY'S TIP: Switch things up! Top the polenta with my Easy Mango Chutney (page 191) or Slow Cooker Cranberry Sauce (page 190).

Serving size: 2 polenta rounds plus 2 tablespoons salsa

Per serving: Calories: 110; Total fat: 5g; Saturated fat: 1g; Protein: 2g; Carbohydrates: 14g; Fiber: 1g; Sodium: 387mg

Sorghum with Mushrooms

GLUTEN-FREE | DAIRY-FREE | PALEO-FRIENDLY | VEGAN | VEGETARIAN

Growing up, I never liked mushrooms, but my mother put them in everything. Finally, as an adult, I became a mushroom fan. I've grown to love mushrooms, especially in grain dishes, just like mom used to feed me when I was a girl.

SERVES 4

FREEZER-FRIENDLY

Prep time: 15 minutes

Cook time: 35 minutes

1 tablespoon olive oil

1 onion, chopped

1 garlic clove, minced

8 ounces baby bella mushrooms, thinly sliced

1 cup pearled sorghum

3 cups low-sodium vegetable broth

¼ cup chopped fresh flat-leaf parsley

¼ teaspoon salt

⅛ teaspoon freshly ground black pepper

1. In a medium saucepan over medium heat, heat the olive oil. Add the onion and cook until translucent, about 3 minutes. Add the garlic and cook until fragrant, 1 minute. Add the mushrooms and cook until softened, about 5 minutes.

2. Add the sorghum and vegetable broth, and bring to a boil. Reduce heat, cover, and simmer, stirring occasionally, for about 25 minutes, until the sorghum becomes puffed and softens.

3. Add the parsley, salt, and pepper, and toss to combine.

4. To freeze, store sorghum in a freezer-safe container in the freezer for up to 2 months. To defrost, refrigerate overnight. Reheat individual portions in the microwave on high for 1 to 2 minutes. To reheat on the stovetop, reheat the entire batch in a saucepan over medium heat for about 5 to 8 minutes, until heated through. Add a splash of liquid if reheating on stovetop.

TOBY'S TIP: Look for sorghum at your local market or online. You can also swap it out for quinoa, farro, brown rice, or barley.

Serving size: 1 cup
Per serving: Calories: 234; Total fat: 5g; Saturated fat: 1g; Protein: 8g; Carbohydrates: 44g; Fiber: 5g; Sodium: 262mg

Black Beans and Farro

Farro is an Italian-born grain that dates back to ancient Rome and is a relative of wheat. One cup of cooked farro has 220 calories, 5 grams of fiber, and 8 grams of protein. It's also brimming with antioxidant vitamins A and E, iron, and potassium. Farro cooks in a one-to-three ratio of grain to liquid and is ready in about 30 minutes.

SERVES 6

FREEZER-FRIENDLY

Prep time: 10 minutes

Cook time: 35 minutes

1 cup farro, rinsed

3 cups low-sodium vegetable broth

1 tablespoon olive oil

1 onion, finely chopped

1 garlic clove, minced

1 (15-ounce) can low-sodium black beans, drained

1 teaspoon ground cumin

¼ teaspoon salt

⅛ teaspoon freshly ground black pepper

1. In a medium pot, bring the farro and broth to a boil. Reduce heat to medium-low and simmer for about 30 minutes, until farro is cooked through. Drain the excess liquid.

2. In a medium skillet over medium heat, heat the olive oil. Add the onion and cook until translucent, about 3 minutes. Add the garlic and cook until fragrant, 1 minute.

3. Add the beans and the cooked farro, and toss until heated through, about 1 minute. Add the cumin, salt, and pepper, and stir to combine.

4. Serve warm or freeze for later. To freeze, allow to cool for 20 to 30 minutes, then place into a resealable freezer-friendly container and freeze for up to 2 months. To defrost, refrigerate overnight. Reheat individual portions, covered, in the microwave for 1 to 2 minutes.

TOBY'S TIP: For a gluten-free version, substitute brown rice, sorghum, quinoa, or millet for the farro.

Serving size: About ¾ cup
Per serving: Calories: 238; Total fat: 4g; Saturated fat: 0g; Protein: 10g; Carbohydrates: 40g; Fiber: 11g; Sodium: 268mg

Pineapple-Cashew Quinoa

GLUTEN-FREE | DAIRY-FREE | VEGAN | VEGETARIAN

When I was growing up, my mom always seemed to make savory dishes sweeter by adding dried or fresh fruit to sides like rice, green salads, and stuffing. As I grew up, I experimented with putting fresh, dried, and canned fruit in my sides, and it's a delicious hack I now use regularly. Plus, it's a fun way to add fruit into lunch or dinner.

SERVES 6

30-MINUTE

Prep time: 10 minutes

Cook time: 20 minutes

1 cup quinoa

2 cups water

1 tablespoon olive oil

1 cup canned pineapple chunks packed in own juice, juice reserved

¼ cup raw unsalted cashews, chopped

½ teaspoon salt

¼ teaspoon freshly ground black pepper

⅛ teaspoon ground nutmeg

1. In a medium saucepan over high heat, bring the quinoa and water to a boil. Reduce heat to low, cover, and simmer for 12 to 15 minutes, until all the liquid has been absorbed. Remove from heat and fluff the quinoa with a fork.

2. In a medium skillet over medium-low heat, heat the olive oil. Add the cooked quinoa, pineapple (reserving the juice), and cashews. Cook, stirring, until heated through, about 3 minutes.

3. Add the reserved pineapple juice, salt, pepper, and nutmeg, and cook until the flavors are combined, an additional 2 minutes.

TOBY'S TIP: Buy too many nuts? Store the extras in a resealable plastic bag in the freezer to make them last longer.

Serving size: About ¾ cup
Per serving: Calories: 247; Total fat: 9g; Saturated fat: 2g; Protein: 6g; Carbohydrates: 37g; Fiber: 3g; Sodium: 106mg

Buffalo Chicken Skewers

GLUTEN-FREE

My kids love spicy chicken skewers, so I decided to make my own at home. My better-for-you combination uses much less butter and is not breaded and fried like many traditional versions. Even better, my kids can't get enough!

SERVES 4

Prep time: 10 minutes, plus 30 minutes to chill

Cook time: 15 minutes

Equipment: 8 wooden skewers

¼ cup hot sauce

1 tablespoon unsalted butter

1 garlic clove, minced

8 pieces (about 14 ounces) chicken tenders

Cooking spray

½ cup Better-for-You Blue Cheese Dressing (page 180)

1. In a small pan over medium heat, heat the hot sauce, butter, and garlic until the butter has melted and the ingredients are combined. Remove from heat and allow to cool for 5 minutes.

2. Place the chicken tenders in a medium bowl. Add the hot sauce mixture and toss to evenly coat.

3. Cover and refrigerate for at least 30 minutes or up to overnight.

4. Thread 1 chicken tender per skewer.

5. Coat a grill pan with cooking spray and heat over medium-high heat. Add the chicken skewers and cook for 10 to 12 minutes, turning once, until the chicken reaches an internal temperature of 165°F.

6. Serve with the dressing on the side.

TOBY'S TIP: Soak the wooden skewers for 20 to 30 minutes before threading.

Serving size: 2 chicken skewers plus 2 tablespoons dressing
Per serving: Calories: 193; Total fat: 7g; Saturated fat: 4g; Protein: 28g; Carbohydrates: 2g; Fiber: 0g; Sodium: 356mg

Roasted Zucchini Boats with Ground Beef

GLUTEN-FREE

Over the years, I've thrown a ton of parties, sometimes with more than 100 guests. For each event, I insist on cooking the food, including killer appetizers like this one. Without fail, at the end of every party, someone asks for this recipe.

SERVES 8

Prep time: 15 minutes

Cook time: 35 minutes

Cooking spray

4 medium zucchini

1 tablespoon olive oil

4 ounces cremini mushrooms, diced

2 garlic cloves, minced

8 ounces 90% lean ground beef

½ cup Basic Tomato Sauce (page 184) or jarred tomato sauce

¼ teaspoon salt

⅛ teaspoon freshly ground black pepper

½ cup shredded part-skim mozzarella cheese

1. Preheat the oven to 350°F. Coat a baking dish with cooking spray.

2. Halve the zucchini lengthwise and, using a teaspoon, scoop out the seeds. Arrange the zucchini halves in the prepared baking dish, leaving space between each zucchini.

3. In a large sauté pan or skillet over medium heat, heat the olive oil. Add the mushrooms and sauté until softened, about 3 minutes. Add the garlic and cook until fragrant, an additional 1 minute.

4. Add the ground beef and cook for 5 minutes, until browned, breaking up the pieces. Add the tomato sauce, salt, and pepper, and stir to combine. Continue cooking for about 3 minutes, until the mixture is heated through. Remove from heat and allow to cool for about 10 minutes.

5. Spoon 2 heaping tablespoons of beef mixture into each zucchini boat, and top each boat with 1 tablespoon of shredded mozzarella.

6. Bake for 20 minutes, until the zucchini are tender and the cheese has melted.

TOBY'S TIP: Keep 1 or 2 jars of store-bought tomato sauce in your pantry to use when you don't have time to make your own. When purchasing, compare labels and look for brands with less added sugar and sodium per serving.

Serving size: 1 zucchini boat
Per serving: Calories: 97; Total fat: 5g; Saturated fat: 2g; Protein: 9g; Carbohydrates: 5g; Fiber: 1g; Sodium: 155mg

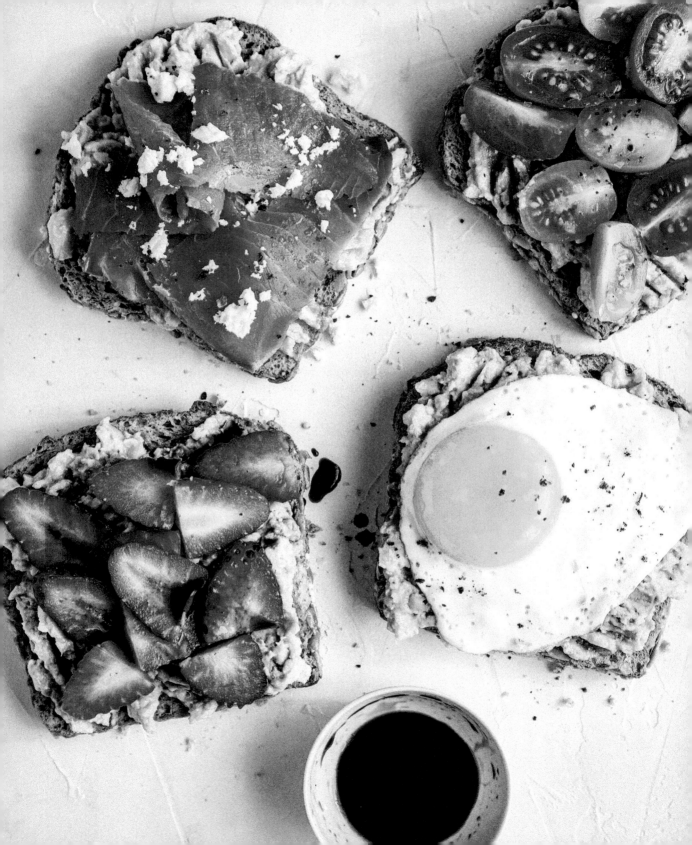

5 Simple Snacks and Mini-Meals

Spiced Popcorn

GLUTEN-FREE | DAIRY-FREE | VEGAN | VEGETARIAN

Family movie night has become a regular activity in my house. I usually try to select kid-friendly movies from when I was growing up that I *need* to have my kids watch. Remember *Parenthood, Cheaper by the Dozen, Sixteen Candles, Grease*? Every movie night is accompanied by a few bowls of popcorn, like this one.

SERVES 4

30-MINUTE

Prep time: 5 minutes

Cook time: 5 minutes

3 tablespoons olive oil

½ cup popcorn kernels

Cooking spray

1 teaspoon garlic powder

1 teaspoon onion powder

½ teaspoon smoked paprika

½ teaspoon salt

⅛ teaspoon cayenne pepper

1. In a medium pot over medium-low heat, heat the olive oil. Add 3 popcorn kernels, and when one of the kernels pops, add the rest. Cover and shake the pot occasionally to prevent burning. Once fully popped, transfer the popcorn to a large bowl.

2. Spray the popcorn with cooking spray. Use clean hands to toss the popcorn, mixing it thoroughly.

3. In a small bowl, mix together the garlic powder, onion powder, paprika, salt, and cayenne.

4. Sprinkle the spice mix over the popcorn, and toss until the popcorn is thoroughly coated.

TOBY'S TIP: A large order of movie theater popcorn can have upward of 1,000 calories and 60 grams of fat! Instead, bag your own spiced popcorn and bring it to the theater. You can also pop the corn for this recipe in an air popper—no oil required.

Serving size: About 4 cups
Per serving: Calories: 175; Total fat: 11g; Saturated fat: 1g; Protein: 3g; Carbohydrates: 19g; Fiber: 4g; Sodium: 295mg

Baked Spinach Chips

GLUTEN-FREE | DAIRY-FREE | PALEO-FRIENDLY | VEGAN | VEGETARIAN

In my first cookbook, *The Greek Yogurt Kitchen*, I include a simple recipe for kale chips. To this day, my daughters love kale chips and devour them every time I bake up a batch. Although I love kale chips, too, I wanted an alternative that would still be a healthy green vegetable my girls would love. After running through my test kitchen with these babies, I'm happy to report that my 10-year-old now requests these spinach chips as her school snack.

SERVES 4

30-MINUTE

Prep time: 5 minutes

Cook time: 15 minutes

Cooking spray

5 ounces baby spinach, washed and patted dry

2 tablespoons olive oil

1 teaspoon garlic powder

½ teaspoon salt

⅛ teaspoon freshly ground black pepper

1. Preheat the oven to 350°F. Coat two baking sheets with cooking spray.

2. Place the spinach in a large bowl. Add the olive oil, garlic powder, salt, and pepper, and toss until evenly coated.

3. Spread the spinach in a single layer on the baking sheets. Bake for 12 to 15 minutes, until the spinach leaves are crisp and slightly browned.

4. Store spinach chips in a resealable container at room temperature for up to 1 week.

TOBY'S TIP: Keep your spice drawer current. Ground spices (like garlic powder) and dried herbs stay fresh up to 1 year, while whole spices can last up to 2 years. To ensure your spices stay as flavorful as possible, store them in a cool, dry place away from heat and sunlight.

Serving size: About ⅔ cup
Per serving: Calories: 77; Total fat: 7g; Saturated fat: 1g; Protein: 1g; Carbohydrates: 4g; Fiber: 2g; Sodium: 351mg

Peanut Butter Yogurt Dip with Fruit

GLUTEN-FREE | VEGETARIAN

Studies show that kids are more likely to eat their fruits and veggies if they get to dip them. I believe the same theory applies for adults, too, especially when the dip is made from delicious and nutritious ingredients!

SERVES 4

ONE POT/ONE PAN

30-MINUTE

Prep time: 10 minutes

1 cup nonfat vanilla
Greek yogurt

2 tablespoons natural
creamy peanut butter

2 teaspoons honey

1 pear, cored and sliced

1 apple, cored and sliced

1 banana, sliced

1. In a medium bowl, whisk together the yogurt, peanut butter, and honey.

2. Serve the dip with the fruit on the side.

TOBY'S TIP: Make a delicious parfait by layering diced fruit with 2 (¼-cup) layers of this dip.

Serving size: ¼ cup dip plus about ¼ cup fruit
Per serving: Calories: 175; Total fat: 4g; Saturated fat: 1g; Protein: 8g; Carbohydrates: 29g; Fiber: 4g; Sodium: 58mg

Snickerdoodle Pecans

GLUTEN-FREE | DAIRY-FREE | VEGAN | VEGETARIAN

I love snacking on nuts and am especially a fan of sweet-flavored nuts. I find, however, that many packaged nuts and DIY recipes are overflowing with added sugar. Although some added sugar is needed to get that sweet flavor, when I make my own, I control the ingredients—especially the added sugar.

SERVES 8

30-MINUTE

Prep time: 10 minutes

Cook time: 15 minutes

Cooking spray

1½ cups raw pecans

2 tablespoons brown sugar

2 tablespoons 100% maple syrup

½ teaspoon ground cinnamon

½ teaspoon vanilla extract

⅛ teaspoon salt

1. Preheat the oven to 350°F. Line a baking sheet with parchment paper and coat with cooking spray.

2. In a medium bowl, place the pecans. Add the brown sugar, maple syrup, cinnamon, vanilla, and salt, tossing to evenly coat.

3. Spread the pecans in a single layer on the prepared baking sheet. Bake for about 12 minutes, until pecans are slightly browned and fragrant. Remove and set aside to cool for 10 minutes.

TOBY'S TIP: Store pecans in an airtight container. If you want to prolong the life of your pecans, you can freeze them. The quality of pecans is not affected by freezing, even if you thaw and refreeze them several times!

Serving size: ¼ cup

Per serving: Calories: 151; Total fat: 13g; Saturated fat: 1g; Protein: 2g; Carbohydrates: 8g; Fiber: 2g; Sodium: 38mg

Almond-Stuffed Dates

GLUTEN-FREE | DAIRY-FREE | PALEO-FRIENDLY | VEGAN | VEGETARIAN

When my son was a toddler, he loved his green vegetables but wouldn't eat most fruits. Dates were the only fruit he would eat, and only if they were stuffed with almonds. The moral of the story is to never give up with picky eaters. They may surprise you with the foods they'll accept. To this day, my son still prefers vegetables over fruits, and he still enjoys almond-stuffed dates.

SERVES 4

30-MINUTE

Prep time: 5 minutes

20 raw almonds

20 pitted dates

Place one almond into each of 20 dates. Serve at room temperature.

TOBY'S TIP: Swap the almonds for pecans, cashews, pistachios, or walnuts.

Serving size: 5 pieces
Per serving: Calories: 137; Total fat: 3g; Saturated fat: 0g; Protein: 2g; Carbohydrates: 28g; Fiber: 4g; Sodium: 1mg

Peanut Butter Chocolate Chip Energy Bites

GLUTEN-FREE | DAIRY-FREE | VEGETARIAN

Snacks are mini-meals, so it's a great idea to include foods and nutrients you may have missed out on during your regular meals. I recommend aiming for up to 200 calories per snack and to make sure they have whole grains, protein, and/or healthy fat to help keep you satisfied. These energy bites are not only scrumptious (what isn't with chocolate and peanut butter?), but they also contain whole-grain oats and healthy unsaturated fat from the peanut butter.

SERVES 12

Prep time: 20 minutes, plus 15 minutes to chill

Cook time: 5 minutes

1 cup gluten-free old-fashioned oats

¾ cup natural creamy peanut butter

½ cup unsweetened coconut flakes

½ teaspoon vanilla extract

2 tablespoons honey

¼ cup dark chocolate chips

1. Preheat the oven to 350°F. Line a baking sheet with parchment paper.

2. Spread the oats on the prepared baking sheet. Bake for 5 minutes, until the oats are browned. Remove from the oven, and set aside to cool for 5 minutes.

3. In a food processor or blender, add the oats, peanut butter, coconut, vanilla, and honey. Blend until smooth.

4. Transfer the batter into a medium bowl, and fold in the chocolate chips.

5. Spoon out a tablespoon of batter. Use clean hands to roll into a 2-inch ball, and place on the baking sheet. Repeat for the remaining batter, making a total of 12 balls.

6. Place the baking sheet in the refrigerator to allow the bites to set, at least 15 minutes.

TOBY'S TIP: To switch up the flavors, swap the chocolate chips with raisins or other dried fruits, such as chopped apricots, cranberries, or tart cherries.

Serving size: 1 piece
Per serving: Calories: 177; Total fat: 12g; Saturated fat: 4g; Protein: 5g; Carbohydrates: 14g; Fiber: 2g; Sodium: 58mg

No-Cook Pistachio-Cranberry Quinoa Bites

Pistachios bring back memories of my childhood growing up in Brooklyn, where my grandfather used to own several Smoke & Reads at Kings Plaza, the local mall. Every time I visited his store, I asked for the red pistachios, which I later found out were dyed. This also explains why my hands and face became stained cherry red every time I ate them. Only as a teenager did I realize the true earthy color of pistachios, but I still love them as much as ever.

SERVES 12

30-MINUTE

Prep time: 15 minutes, plus 15 minutes to chill

½ cup quinoa

¾ cup natural almond butter

¾ cup gluten-free old-fashioned oats

2 tablespoons honey

⅛ teaspoon salt

¼ cup unsalted shelled pistachios, roughly chopped

¼ cup dried cranberries

1. In a blender, add the quinoa and blend until it turns into a flour consistency.

2. Add the almond butter, oats, honey, and salt, and blend until smooth.

3. Transfer the mixture into a medium bowl, and gently fold in the pistachios and cranberries.

4. Spoon out a tablespoon of the batter. Use clean hands to roll into a 2-inch ball, and place into a container. Repeat for the remaining batter, making a total of 12 balls.

5. Place the container in the refrigerator to allow the bites to set, at least 15 minutes.

TOBY'S TIP: Although you may be used to seeing pistachios in the shell, you can now find shelled pistachios at your local market, which work beautifully over salads; in baked goods, like muffins and cookies; and in these bites.

Serving size: 1 piece
Per serving: Calories: 175; Total fat: 11g; Saturated fat: 1g; Protein: 6g; Carbohydrates: 16g; Fiber: 3g; Sodium: 25mg

No-Bake Honey-Almond Granola Bars

Many of the "old-school" granola bars, like the ones my mom used to pack for me for the bus ride home, contain lots of preservatives and added sugar. I am also rather selective with the bars that I choose today; although they may have better-for-you ingredients, not all are tasty. Luckily, I DIY my granola bars to make them both tasty and full of the ingredients I want.

SERVES 8

Prep time: 15 minutes, plus 1 to 2 hours to chill

Cooking spray

1 cup pitted dates

¼ cup honey

¾ cup natural creamy almond butter

¾ cup gluten-free rolled oats

2 tablespoons raw almonds, chopped

2 tablespoons pumpkin seeds

1. Line an 8-by-8-inch baking dish with parchment paper, and coat the paper with cooking spray.

2. In a food processor or blender, add the dates and blend until they reach a pastelike consistency. Add the honey, almond butter, and oats, and blend until well combined. Transfer the mixture to a medium bowl.

3. Add the almonds and pumpkin seeds, and gently fold until well combined.

4. Spoon the mixture into the prepared baking dish. Spread the mixture evenly, using clean fingers to push down the mixture so it is compact.

5. Cover with plastic wrap and refrigerate until the bars set, 1 to 2 hours.

6. Remove from the refrigerator and cut into 8 bars. Carefully remove each bar from the baking dish, and wrap individually in plastic wrap. Place bars in the refrigerator until ready to grab and go.

TOBY'S TIP: Swap the honey for 100% maple syrup to make these bars vegan.

Serving size: 1 bar
Per serving: Calories: 296; Total fat: 16g; Saturated fat: 0g; Protein: 8g; Carbohydrates: 32g; Fiber: 5g; Sodium: 1mg

Cottage Cheese–Filled Avocado

GLUTEN-FREE | VEGETARIAN

Want to try something unique? Pair the most appreciated fruit with the most under-appreciated dairy food, and you'll get one of the tastiest, healthiest snacks in just 5 minutes.

SERVES 4

ONE POT/ONE PAN
30-MINUTE

Prep time: 5 minutes

½ cup low-fat cottage cheese

¼ cup cherry tomatoes, quartered

2 avocados, halved and pitted

4 teaspoons pumpkin seeds

¼ teaspoon salt

⅛ teaspoon freshly ground black pepper

1. In a small bowl, mix together the cottage cheese and tomatoes.

2. Spoon 2 tablespoons of the cheese-tomato mixture onto each of the avocado halves. Top each with 1 teaspoon of pumpkin seeds, and sprinkle with the salt and pepper.

TOBY'S TIP: You can make this avocado dairy-free by swapping the cottage cheese for a chopped hardboiled egg, salsa, or tuna salad.

Serving size: 1 avocado half
Per serving: Calories: 197; Total fat: 16g; Saturated fat: 3g; Protein: 6g; Carbohydrates: 10g; Fiber: 7g; Sodium: 270mg

Avocado Toast with Balsamic Glaze

DAIRY-FREE | VEGAN | VEGETARIAN

Avocado toast is so popular that some restaurants now have it on the menu. Instead of paying $10 for an order, you can make your own. Start with a simple avocado-tomato combo, and once you've mastered it, move on to more creative additions, like beans and sriracha, fried egg, sliced strawberries, or smoked salmon and crumbled feta.

SERVES 2

**ONE POT/ONE PAN
30-MINUTE**

Prep time: 5 minutes
Cook time: 10 minutes

¼ cup balsamic vinegar

1 tablespoon brown sugar

1 ripe avocado, halved and pitted

2 slices 100% whole-wheat bread, toasted

5 cherry tomatoes, halved

⅛ teaspoon salt

⅛ teaspoon freshly ground black pepper

1. In a small saucepan over medium heat, heat the vinegar and brown sugar, stirring constantly, until the sugar dissolves. Bring the mixture to a boil, lower heat, and simmer for about 10 minutes, until the vinegar is reduced by half and thickens. Set aside to cool for 10 minutes.

2. Scoop out the flesh from each avocado half onto a slice of toasted bread. Mash the avocado with a fork until it is flattened.

3. Top each slice of bread with 5 tomato halves, and sprinkle with the salt and pepper.

4. Drizzle about ½ tablespoon of the balsamic glaze on each avocado toast.

TOBY'S TIP: You can make a glaze using 100% pomegranate juice. Heat the juice over medium heat until it reaches a boil. Then lower heat and simmer until the juice is reduced by half and becomes so thick it sticks to the bottom of a spoon. It's a tasty alternative to balsamic glaze that you can use on chicken, fish, and avocado toast.

Serving size: 1 avocado toast
Per serving: Calories: 292; Total fat: 16g; Saturated fat: 2g; Protein: 7g; Carbohydrates: 33g; Fiber: 10g; Sodium: 289mg

Whole-Wheat Chocolate-Banana "Quesadillas"

This sweet snack is a spinoff of a hazelnut spread–banana crêpe I went crazy over in Paris. Instead of making crêpes, I use whole-wheat tortillas and swap out the nut butters and fruit upon request.

SERVES 4

30-MINUTE

Prep time: 5 minutes
Cook time: 5 minutes

Cooking spray

2 (10-inch) whole-wheat tortillas

1½ ounces 60% dark chocolate

2 tablespoons natural creamy peanut butter

1 medium banana, thinly sliced

1. Heat a medium skillet coated with cooking spray over medium heat. Add a tortilla and warm for 30 seconds on each side. Place the warmed tortilla on a plate, and repeat with the second tortilla.

2. In a small bowl, melt the chocolate in the microwave, about 1 minute, stirring halfway through.

3. Using a spatula, spread the peanut butter onto 1 tortilla to the edges. Top with the banana slices, and drizzle the chocolate over the peanut butter.

4. Top with the second tortilla, pressing down gently with the palm of your hand.

5. Cut into 8 pieces and serve.

TOBY'S TIP: Other favorite combinations include almond butter and pears, walnut butter and blueberries, and peanut butter and unsweetened coconut flakes, with or without a drizzle of dark chocolate or chocolate hazelnut spread.

Serving size: 2 pieces
Per serving: Calories: 225; Total fat: 12g; Saturated fat: 4g; Protein: 6g; Carbohydrates: 28g; Fiber: 5g; Sodium: 289mg

Whole-Grain Mexican-Style Roll-Ups

VEGETARIAN

I spent many summers in Israel, where dinner is usually cereal and milk or an omelet. As such, I prefer a small dinner or enjoy a mini-meal, like my Green Shakshuka (page 90) or these bite-size roll-ups. I pair this dish with cut-up vegetables or a small salad to make it even more filling.

SERVES 4

Prep time: 10 minutes, plus 1 to 2 hours to chill

½ cup nonfat plain Greek yogurt

½ cup reduced-fat sour cream

¼ teaspoon salt

⅛ teaspoon freshly ground black pepper

1 cup shredded pepper Jack cheese

1 (15-ounce) can low-sodium black beans, drained, rinsed, and mashed

2 (10-inch) whole-wheat tortillas

1. In a medium bowl, mix together the yogurt, sour cream, salt, and pepper. Stir in the cheese and mashed beans.

2. Lay the tortillas side by side on a cutting board. Spread 1 cup of the mixture onto each tortilla out to the edges.

3. Roll up each tortilla and cut off the uneven ends. Wrap each in plastic wrap and refrigerate for 1 to 2 hours.

4. Remove from the refrigerator and cut each into 8 (1-inch) roll-ups.

TOBY'S TIP: When mixing Greek yogurt with a condiment, like sour cream, mayo, or cream cheese, I like using equal amounts of both. I love the taste of these condiments, which still shines through when I use my one-to-one yogurt-to-condiment ratio.

Serving size: 4 pieces
Per serving: Calories: 323; Total fat: 16g; Saturated fat: 8g; Protein 18g; Carbohydrates: 32g; Fiber: 8g; Sodium: 817mg

Chicken Nacho Bites

GLUTEN-FREE

There's no way I'm serving my guests or kids nachos with that fake movie theater or bowling alley cheese! My hearty, mouthwatering nachos are made with heart-healthy beans, protein-packed chicken, and calcium-rich cheese. Top that, fake cheese stuff!

SERVES 4

30-MINUTE

Prep time: 15 minutes

Cook time: 10 minutes

Cooking spray

¾ cup low-sodium black beans, drained and rinsed

½ teaspoon hot sauce

¼ teaspoon salt

20 corn tortilla chips

3 ounces Easy Sautéed Chicken Breast (page 118) or rotisserie chicken, coarsely chopped into 20 bite-size pieces

½ cup shredded reduced-fat sharp Cheddar cheese

1. Preheat the oven to 400°F. Coat two baking sheets with cooking spray.

2. In a medium bowl, add the beans, hot sauce, and salt, and toss to combine. Using a masher or the back of a fork, coarsely mash.

3. Spread the tortilla chips on the prepared baking sheets. Top each chip with 1 teaspoon of the black bean mixture, 1 piece of chicken, and 1 teaspoon of cheese.

4. Bake for 5 to 7 minutes, until the cheese has melted.

TOBY'S TIP: Add some more healthy ingredients to these nachos— try jalapeño slices and Simple Salsa (page 189).

Serving size: 5 pieces

Per serving: Calories: 185; Total fat: 7g; Saturated fat: 2g; Protein: 14g; Carbohydrates: 18g; Fiber: 4g; Sodium: 388mg

Snack Pizza with Chicken and Mushrooms

Pizza can be less than healthy depending on the ingredients, but if you make it at home, you have control over what goes on it. My snack pizza provides four food groups, including whole grains, dairy, vegetables, and protein. It's a quick and easy snack that is filling and makes me feel like I'm getting the nourishment my body needs. My kids, too, can't seem to get enough, so it's a go-to snack I have been serving up for years.

SERVES 4

30-MINUTE

Prep time: 10 minutes

Cook time: 10 minutes

Cooking spray

6 button mushrooms, chopped

3 ounces Easy Sautéed Chicken Breast (page 118) or leftover chicken, chopped into bite-size pieces

4 whole-wheat English muffins

1 cup Basic Tomato Sauce (page 184) or jarred tomato sauce

½ cup shredded part-skim mozzarella cheese

1. Preheat the oven to 350°F. Coat a baking sheet with cooking spray.

2. In a small bowl, toss together the mushrooms and chicken.

3. Split each of the English muffins and place crust-side down on the prepared baking sheet, leaving about 1 inch between them. Top each with 2 tablespoons of Basic Tomato Sauce (page 184), and using the back of the spoon, spread the sauce to the edges of the bread. Top the tomato sauce with 3 tablespoons of the mushroom-chicken mixture, then 1 tablespoon of cheese.

4. Bake for about 10 minutes, until the cheese has melted and the bread is slightly toasted.

5. Remove from the oven and allow to cool for 10 minutes before serving.

TOBY'S TIP: To make the pizza vegetarian, swap the chicken for beans or vegetables, like peppers and onions. To make this dish gluten-free, use your favorite gluten-free bread or gluten-free English muffin (I like Mikey's Muffins).

Serving size: 2 pizzas

Per serving: Calories: 220; Total fat: 5g; Saturated fat: 2g; Protein: 17g; Carbohydrates: 29g; Fiber: 4g; Sodium: 666mg

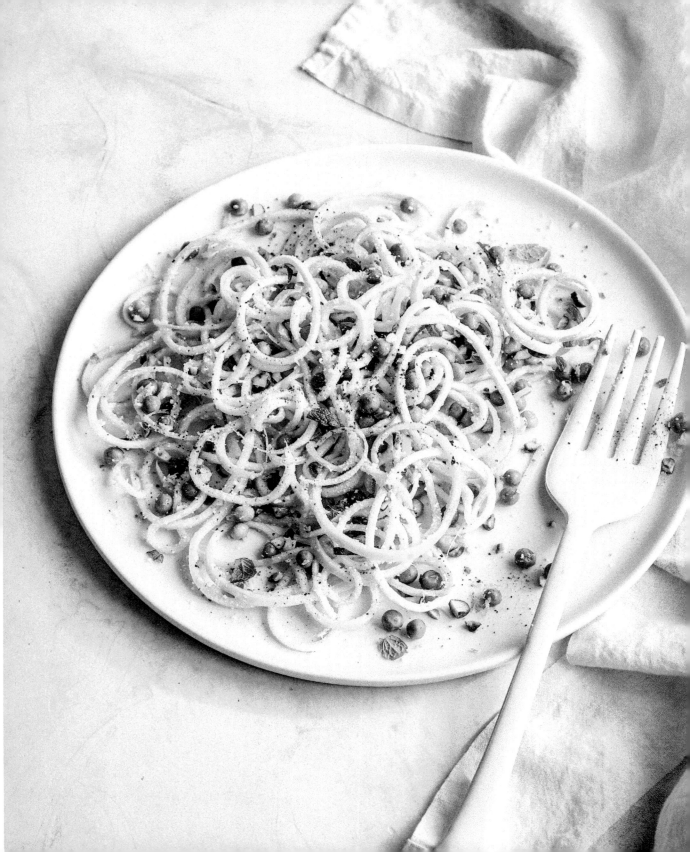

6 Vegan and Vegetarian Mains

Cheesy Lentil-Spinach Quesadillas

My absolute go-to meal any time of the day is quesadillas. I can fill them up with eggs and beans for breakfast or leftover chili or veggies, like in this simple vegetarian version, for dinner. I even pack a basic cheese quesadilla in my 10-year-old's lunch box. The possibilities are endless, and I have such a fun time experimenting with different foods to mix and match.

SERVES 4

30-MINUTE

Prep time: 10 minutes

Cook time: 20 minutes

Cooking spray

1 tablespoon olive oil

1 onion, chopped

1 (15-ounce) can low-sodium lentils, drained and rinsed

8 cups (about 6 ounces) shredded spinach

¼ teaspoon salt

¼ teaspoon freshly ground black pepper

8 (8-inch) whole-wheat tortillas

1 cup shredded reduced-fat sharp Cheddar cheese

1. Preheat the oven to 400°F. Coat two baking sheets with cooking spray.

2. In a medium skillet over medium heat, heat the olive oil. Add the onion and cook until translucent, about 3 minutes. Add the lentils and cook until heated through, about 2 minutes. Add half the spinach and cook until it begins to wilt, about 3 minutes, then add the second half of the spinach and continue cooking until all the spinach is wilted, about 4 more minutes. Add the salt and pepper, and toss to combine.

3. Coat one side of 4 tortillas with cooking spray, and place 2 tortillas coated-side down on each baking sheet. Divide the lentil mixture evenly between the 4 tortillas, and using the back of a spoon, spread it to the edges of the tortillas. Sprinkle each tortilla with ¼ cup of cheese, and top with another tortilla. Use clean hands to gently press down with your palm on each quesadilla.

4. Bake for 8 minutes, until the cheese has melted and the tortillas are slightly browned.

5. Remove from the oven and allow to cool for 5 minutes. Slice each quesadilla into 4 quarters and serve.

TOBY'S TIP: To make this dish for meat eaters, add a few ounces of leftover chicken to the lentil mixture. Both versions can be served with Simple Salsa (page 189).

Serving size: 1 quesadilla

Per serving: Calories: 447; Total fat: 16g; Saturated fat: 7g; Protein: 21g; Carbohydrates: 56g; Fiber: 17g; Sodium: 897mg

Yellow Squash Noodles with Peas and Mint

GLUTEN-FREE | VEGETARIAN

A few years ago, my sister bought me a spiralizer as a housewarming gift. I was daunted by the idea of assembling it and dismissed the idea of adding another kitchen tool to my collection. One day, I decided to see what my spiralizer could do and whipped it out from the back of the pantry. I assembled it in two minutes, and then started spiralizing all kinds of goodies—apples, cucumbers, squash, carrots, pears, and even parsnips. Oh, the fun I had playing (and eating) using my new toy!

SERVES 4

30-MINUTE

Prep time: 15 minutes
Cook time: 5 minutes
Equipment: Spiralizer

1 cup frozen peas

3 medium yellow squash, or 6 cups precut squash noodles

½ cup chopped fresh mint

2 garlic cloves, minced

Zest and juice of 1 lemon

3 tablespoons olive oil

⅛ teaspoon freshly ground black pepper

¾ cup grated Parmesan cheese

½ cup raw shelled pistachios, chopped

1. In a small saucepan, bring 1 cup of water to a boil. Add the frozen peas, reduce heat, and simmer until heated through, about 5 minutes. Drain and allow the peas to cool.

2. Using a spiralizer, make the squash noodles and place in a large bowl. Set aside.

3. In another large bowl, whisk the mint, garlic, lemon zest and juice, olive oil, and pepper.

4. Add the peas and squash noodles to the dressing and toss to evenly coat. Add the Parmesan, gently tossing to combine.

5. Sprinkle with the pistachios and serve.

TOBY'S TIP: Swap the squash for zucchini, or spiralize a colorful combo of zucchini and squash. If you don't have a spiralizer, you can look up instructions to use a vegetable peeler, knife, or grater to make the squash noodles.

Serving size: 2 cups
Per serving: Calories: 315; Total fat 23g; Saturated fat: 6g; Protein: 14g; Carbohydrates: 16g; Fiber: 5g; Sodium: 330mg

Baked Lentil Falafel

DAIRY-FREE | VEGAN | VEGETARIAN

When I dine at a Mediterranean restaurant, I don't order falafel balls because they're deep-fried. I'll also skip the frozen kind with all the preservatives and additives. Instead, I whip up my own, but I like to switch around the legume. Some days I use chickpeas, like in traditional falafel, or, like in this recipe, I opt for lentils.

SERVES 4

FREEZER-FRIENDLY

Prep time: 10 minutes

Cook time: 40 minutes

Cooking spray

1 teaspoon olive oil

1 small onion, finely chopped

4 garlic cloves, minced

½ teaspoon ground cumin

¼ teaspoon cayenne pepper

½ cup canned low-sodium red or brown lentils, rinsed and drained

1½ cups water

½ teaspoon salt

¼ cup Homemade Bread Crumbs (page 192) or plain bread crumbs

1. Preheat the oven to 425°F. Coat a baking sheet with cooking spray.

2. In a small saucepan over medium heat, heat the olive oil. Add the onion and cook until translucent, 3 minutes. Add the garlic, cumin, cayenne, and lentils, and cook through for 1 minute.

3. Add the water and bring the mixture to a boil. Reduce heat and simmer until all the water is absorbed, about 15 minutes. Remove from heat and set aside to cool for 10 minutes.

4. Add the salt and bread crumbs, and stir until the mixture is smooth.

5. Spoon out 1 tablespoon of the mixture. Use clean hands to roll into a ball, then flatten into a ½-inch-thick disk. Repeat for a total of 12 disks. Place them on the prepared baking sheet, leaving about 1 inch between each.

6. Bake for 15 minutes, then flip them and bake for an additional 5 minutes.

7. Remove from the oven and allow to cool for 10 minutes before serving. To freeze, place cooled falafel into a resealable freezer-safe container in the freezer for up to 2 months. To defrost, refrigerate overnight. Reheat in a 350°F oven for 10 minutes. Alternatively, reheat several pieces in the microwave on high for about 1 minute.

TOBY'S TIP: Serve with Tahini Yogurt Sauce (page 186), or stuff into whole-wheat pitas together with Mediterranean Chopped Salad (page 41) and a spoonful of hummus.

Serving size: 3 pieces

Per serving: Calories: 155; Total fat: 4g; Saturated fat: 1g; Protein: 8g; Carbohydrates: 22g; Fiber: 4g; Sodium: 351mg

Quinoa-Stuffed Acorn Squash

GLUTEN-FREE | DAIRY-FREE | VEGAN | VEGETARIAN

When I was growing up, my mother had every type of squash on our table. From butternut to acorn to spaghetti, she always found a fun way to serve it up. My favorite way, however, was when she stuffed acorn squash with a whole grain combined with dried fruit. In this stuffed acorn squash recipe, the sweet cranberries balance the more bitter kale flavor, which is all rounded out with the quinoa.

SERVES 4

Prep time: 10 minutes

Cook time: 35 minutes

½ cup quinoa

1 cup water

2 medium acorn squash (about 2½ pounds)

1 tablespoon olive oil

1 garlic clove, minced

Zest and juice of 1 lemon

¼ teaspoon salt

⅛ teaspoon freshly ground black pepper

2 cups chopped kale

½ cup dried cranberries

1. In a medium pot, add the quinoa and water, and bring to a boil. Reduce heat and simmer until quinoa is cooked through, about 15 minutes. Fluff the quinoa with a fork.

2. Using a knife, pierce the skin of both squash several times. Place them in a microwave and cook for 18 minutes, rotating each halfway though. Carefully remove the squash from the microwave and place them on a cutting board. Halve both squash lengthwise, and use a spoon to scoop out the seeds.

3. In a medium bowl, whisk the oil, garlic, lemon zest and juice, salt, and pepper. Add the kale, tossing to combine.

4. Add the cooked quinoa and the cranberries to the kale mixture, and stir to combine.

5. Scoop ½ cup of the quinoa mixture into each of the 4 squash halves and serve.

TOBY'S TIP: To cook acorn squash in the oven, halve the squash lengthwise and use a spoon to scoop out the seeds. Place the squash flesh-side down on a baking sheet coated with cooking spray, and bake at 425°F until golden and soft, about 25 minutes.

Serving size: 1 squash half

Per serving: Calories: 286; Total fat: 6g; Saturated fat: 1g; Protein: 7g; Carbohydrates: 57g; Fiber: 8g; Sodium: 173mg

Tofu Stir-Fry with Yellow Peppers

DAIRY-FREE | VEGAN | VEGETARIAN

When I first learned to cook, tofu stir-fry was one of the first dishes I made. I would take whatever leftover ingredients I found in the refrigerator and toss them together with tofu. Once you get the hang of it, you'll find it to be an easy, versatile go-to dish.

SERVES 4

ONE POT/ONE PAN
30-MINUTE

Prep time: 10 minutes

Cook time: 5 minutes

1 tablespoon olive oil

1 (14-ounce) block extra-firm tofu, cut into 12 (1-inch) slices and patted dry

1 yellow bell pepper, seeded and cut into ½-inch strips

1 small onion, cut into ⅛-inch-thick slices

2 garlic cloves, minced

½ cup Soy-Ginger Sauce (page 188)

1. In a wok or heavy-bottomed skillet over high heat, heat the oil.

2. Add the tofu slices and cook until heated through, about 1 minute on each side. Remove from the pan and set aside.

3. Add the pepper and onion to the pan, and cook for about 3 minutes, until the pepper is softened and the onion is translucent. Add the garlic and cook until fragrant, an additional minute. Whisk the Soy-Ginger Sauce, then add it to the pan. Add the tofu and coat with the sauce.

4. Serve warm.

TOBY'S TIP: Serve this stir-fry over quinoa, brown rice, or farro.

Serving size: About 1 cup
Per serving: Calories: 172; Total fat: 12g; Saturated fat: 1g; Protein: 9g; Carbohydrates: 9g; Fiber: 1g; Sodium: 121mg

Green Shakshuka

GLUTEN-FREE | VEGETARIAN

Traditional shakshuka, made with eggs in a tomato sauce, is a favorite choice when I don't want a big dinner (you can find the recipe for Zippy's Shakshuka in my previous cookbook, *The Healthy Meal Prep Cookbook*). This spin on shakshuka uses green leafy veggies, specifically kale and spinach, and is a welcome addition to my shakshuka repertoire. Just watch to make sure the spinach doesn't overwilt when cooking.

SERVES 4

ONE POT/ONE PAN
30-MINUTE

Prep time: 5 minutes

Cook time: 15 minutes

1 tablespoon olive oil

6 cups chopped kale

6 cups chopped spinach

2 garlic cloves, minced

½ cup chopped fresh dill

½ teaspoon salt

⅛ teaspoon freshly ground black pepper

1 cup part-skim ricotta cheese

4 large eggs

1 lemon, quartered

1. In a large skillet over medium heat, heat the oil. Add the kale and spinach, and sauté for 3 to 4 minutes, until the greens begin to wilt. Add the garlic and cook until fragrant, an additional 1 minute. Stir in the dill, salt, and pepper. Reduce heat to medium-low, and add the ricotta, one spoonful at a time, gently folding it into the greens.

2. Using the back of a spoon, make 4 wells in the greens at each corner of the outer edge of the pan.

3. Break 1 egg into a wineglass. Gently pour the egg into one well along the outer edge. Repeat with the remaining 3 eggs. Cover the pan and cook until the eggs are set, about 8 minutes.

4. Serve with lemon wedges.

TOBY'S TIP: Serve with Simple Salsa (page 189) and Mediterranean Chopped Salad (page 41)

Serving size: 1 egg plus ¼ of the greens
Per serving: Calories: 246; Total fat: 14g; Saturated fat: 5g; Protein: 18g; Carbohydrates: 15g; Fiber: 3g; Sodium: 534mg

Black Bean–Quinoa Burgers

GLUTEN-FREE | DAIRY-FREE | VEGETARIAN

When I was studying to become a registered dietitian, I interned at New York Presbyterian Hospital in Park Slope, Brooklyn. For lunch, the cafeteria served veggie burgers, which I would order every day. After I was finished with my internship, I ended up working as a clinical dietitian at the hospital and still ordered the veggie burgers daily. Once I moved on to my new job, I went through vegetarian burger withdrawal and started making my own.

SERVES 4

FREEZER-FRIENDLY

Prep time: 15 minutes

Cook time: 25 minutes

¼ cup quinoa

½ cup water

1 (15-ounce) can low-sodium black beans, drained and rinsed

1 medium carrot, grated

¼ cup gluten-free old-fashioned oats

1 egg, beaten

¼ teaspoon salt

⅛ teaspoon freshly ground black pepper

2 tablespoons olive oil

1. In a medium saucepan over high heat, bring the quinoa and water to a boil. Reduce heat to low, cover, and simmer for 12 to 15 minutes, until all the liquid has been absorbed. Remove from heat, and fluff the quinoa with a fork.

2. Place the black beans in a large bowl and mash with the back of a fork. Add the cooked quinoa, carrot, oats, egg, salt, and pepper, stirring to incorporate.

3. In a large skillet over medium heat, heat the oil.

4. Scoop out ¼ cup of the quinoa mixture, and use clean hands to form into a patty. Gently press down with the palm of your hand to form a disc, and place on a large plate. Repeat 3 more times with the remaining quinoa mixture.

5. When the oil is shimmering, place the patties into the oil, leaving ½ inch between each patty. Cook for about 8 minutes, flipping once, until the burgers are browned and cooked through.

6. Serve warm or freeze. To freeze, place cooled quinoa burgers in a freezer-safe container in the freezer for up to 2 months. To defrost, refrigerate overnight. Reheat one burger at a time in the microwave on high for 1 to 2 minutes. Burgers can also be reheated in a nonstick skillet over medium heat for about 5 minutes, flipping once.

TOBY'S TIP: Switch the black beans with kidney beans or lentils, or use a combination of any or all of them. If you don't mind the dairy, you can also add ¼ cup of grated Parmesan cheese for even more flavor.

Serving size: 1 burger

Per serving: Calories: 258; Total fat: 10g; Saturated fat: 2g; Protein: 11g; Carbohydrates: 32g; Fiber: 10g; Sodium: 324mg

Creole Stuffed Peppers

GLUTEN-FREE | DAIRY-FREE | VEGAN | VEGETARIAN

As you can see, I am a big fan of meal prep and planning ahead. Stuffed peppers are a freezer-friendly dish, so you can make a double batch, enjoy half during the week, and freeze half for a future busy workweek. Other freezer-friendly dishes you'll find in this cookbook include Slow Cooker Two-Bean Chili (page 96), Black Bean-Quinoa Burgers (page 91), Chicken Marsala (page 127), and Slow Cooker Beef with Bell Peppers (page 146), to name just a few.

SERVES 4

FREEZER-FRIENDLY

Prep time: 15 minutes

Cook time: 1 hour 5 minutes

½ cup brown rice

1 cup water

Cooking spray

1 tablespoon olive oil

1 onion, diced

2 garlic cloves, minced

2 teaspoons Creole seasoning

¾ cup Basic Tomato Sauce (page 184) or jarred tomato sauce

¼ teaspoon salt

⅛ teaspoon freshly ground black pepper

4 green bell peppers

1 lemon, quartered

1. In a saucepan over high heat, add the rice and water, and bring to a boil. Reduce heat to medium-low and simmer for about 40 minutes, or until the rice is tender. Alternatively, use a rice cooker to cook the rice. Fluff with a fork and set aside.

2. Preheat the oven to 400°F. Coat a large baking dish with cooking spray.

3. In a medium sauté pan or skillet over medium heat, heat the olive oil. Add the onion and cook until translucent, about 3 minutes. Add the garlic and Creole seasoning, and cook until the garlic is fragrant, an additional 1 minute. Add the cooked brown rice, tomato sauce, salt, and pepper, and toss to combine.

4. Cut off the tops of the bell peppers. Using a paring knife, gently remove the membrane and seeds.

5. Spoon ½ cup of the brown rice mixture into each bell pepper, and arrange the peppers in the prepared baking dish, leaving about 2 inches between each. Cover with aluminum foil and bake for 20 to 25 minutes, until the peppers are soft.

6. Serve each stuffed pepper with a wedge of lemon or freeze for later. To freeze, place cooled peppers in a freezer-safe container in the freezer for up to 2 months. To defrost, refrigerate overnight. Reheat one pepper at a time in the microwave on high for 2 to 3 minutes. Peppers can also be reheated in the oven at 350°F until heated through, 10 to 15 minutes.

TOBY'S TIP: For more protein, add ½ cup cubed extra-firm tofu or beans to the rice.

Serving size: 1 stuffed pepper

Per serving: Calories: 168; Total fat: 4g; Saturated fat: 1g; Protein: 4g; Carbohydrates: 30g; Fiber: 4g; Sodium: 917mg

Tortilla Española with Sweet Potatoes

GLUTEN-FREE | DAIRY-FREE | VEGETARIAN

Sweet potatoes are bursting with nutrition, with one medium potato providing 105 calories and 4 grams of fiber. These babies are also brimming with antioxidant vitamins A and C, potassium, manganese, and the antioxidant lycopene, shown to help fight certain types of cancer and heart disease.

SERVES 4

Prep time: 15 minutes

Cook time: 40 minutes

Cooking spray

1 tablespoon olive oil

1 onion, finely chopped

2 vegetarian bacon slices (about 1 ounce), diced

1 garlic clove, minced

2 sweet potatoes, peeled, halved lengthwise, and cut into ¼-inch-thick pieces (about 3 cups)

2 tablespoons water

8 large eggs

¼ teaspoon salt

⅛ teaspoon freshly ground black pepper

1. Preheat the oven to 350°F. Coat a 6-by-9-inch baking dish with cooking spray.

2. In a medium sauté pan or skillet over medium heat, heat the oil. Add the onion and vegetarian bacon, and gently cook for 5 minutes, stirring occasionally, until the onion is translucent and the bacon is browned. Add the garlic and cook until fragrant, 1 minute. Add the sweet potatoes and toss to combine. Add the water, cover, and cook for 8 minutes, until the potatoes are softened.

3. Carefully pour the mixture into the prepared baking dish, and use the back of a wooden spoon to even out the top.

4. In a medium bowl, whisk the eggs, salt, and pepper. Pour the egg mixture over the potatoes, and bake for 25 to 30 minutes, until the eggs are set.

5. Cut into 4 pieces and serve warm.

TOBY'S TIP: For a meat-eater's or Paleo version, swap the vegetarian bacon for Canadian bacon.

Serving size: 1 piece
Per serving: Calories: 267; Total fat: 14g; Saturated fat: 4g; Protein 16g; Carbohydrates: 20g; Fiber: 3g; Sodium: 447mg

Tofu-Mushroom Ragù over Spaghetti Squash

GLUTEN-FREE | DAIRY-FREE | VEGAN | VEGETARIAN

There's a lot of nutrition packed in those small cremini mushrooms! One cup of sliced mushrooms contains around 20 calories and provides a boatload of nutrients in relation to their total calorie content. Top nutrients include folate, thiamine, vitamin B_6, iron, and zinc. Mushrooms also contain the powerful antioxidant L-ergothioneine, shown to help protect the liver and kidneys.

SERVES 4

Prep time: 15 minutes

Cook time: 35 minutes

1 large spaghetti squash

1 tablespoon olive oil

1 onion, finely chopped

1 pound cremini mushrooms, roughly diced

½ teaspoon salt

2 garlic cloves, minced

1 (28-ounce) can diced tomatoes

1 (14-ounce) package extra-firm tofu, drained and cut into 1-inch cubes

⅛ teaspoon freshly ground black pepper

1. Using a fork, pierce the squash several times on all sides. Place in a microwave, and cook on high for 5 minutes; rotate one-third of the way and cook for another 5; and rotate another one-third and cook for another 5. Remove the squash and allow to cool for 15 minutes.

2. In a large saucepan over medium heat, heat the olive oil. Add the onion and cook, stirring occasionally, until translucent, 3 minutes. Add the mushrooms and salt, and cook, stirring occasionally, until softened, 5 minutes. Add the garlic and cook until fragrant, 1 minute.

3. Stir in the diced tomatoes and bring the mixture to a boil. Reduce heat and simmer until the flavors blend, 5 minutes. Add the tofu and pepper, and toss to evenly coat with the tomato sauce. Continue cooking for 5 minutes, until the tofu is warmed through.

4. Halve the spaghetti squash lengthwise. Use a spoon to scoop out the seeds. Using a fork, scrape the flesh out to create spaghetti-like strands.

5. Distribute the spaghetti squash between 4 bowls, and top each with a quarter of the ragù.

TOBY'S TIP: If spaghetti squash isn't in season, try this mushroom ragù over brown rice, quinoa, whole-grain pasta, or riced cauliflower.

Serving size: About 2 cups
Per serving: Calories: 268; Total fat: 10g; Saturated fat: 1g; Protein: 15g; Carbohydrates: 36g; Fiber: 9g; Sodium: 751mg

Slow Cooker Two-Bean Chili

GLUTEN-FREE | DAIRY-FREE | VEGAN | VEGETARIAN

Warm up on a cold day with this classic comfort food. Full of nutritious ingredients, chili can also be customized to your taste preferences. This vegetarian version uses two different types of beans, though you can also toss in russet or sweet potatoes, or add some heat using hot sauce or sriracha.

SERVES 4

**SLOW COOKER
FREEZER-FRIENDLY**

Prep time: 10 minutes

Cook time: 3 hours on high or
8 hours on low

1 onion, chopped

2 garlic cloves, minced

1 (15-ounce) can low-sodium
black beans, drained
and rinsed

1 (15-ounce) can low-sodium
kidney beans, drained
and rinsed

1½ cups Simple Salsa
(page 189) or jarred salsa

2 cups low-sodium
vegetable broth

½ teaspoon salt

¼ teaspoon freshly
ground black pepper

1. In a slow cooker, add the onion, garlic, black beans, kidney beans, salsa, broth, salt, and pepper. Stir well to combine.

2. Cook on high for 3 hours or on low for 8 hours.

3. Serve warm or freeze for later. To freeze, store cooled chili in individual containers or one large freezer-safe container for up to 2 months. Defrost in the refrigerator overnight. Reheat in the microwave on high for several minutes depending on the portion size, or reheat in a pot over medium-low heat for 10 to 15 minutes.

TOBY'S TIP: Make this a three-bean chili by adding 1 (15-ounce) can of cannellini beans and an additional ½ cup of salsa.

Serving size: 1½ cups
Per serving: Calories: 253; Total fat: 3g; Saturated fat: 0g; Protein: 14g; Carbohydrates: 44g; Fiber: 14g; Sodium: 785mg

Slow Cooker White Bean Stew

GLUTEN-FREE | DAIRY-FREE | VEGAN | VEGETARIAN

Most Americans get less than half the recommended amount of fiber, but beans are an excellent way to get a healthy dose, with 7½ grams per ½-cup serving. This boost of fiber will make you feel full faster and longer. Plus, fiber has been shown to help reduce the risk of colon cancer and contributes to a healthy digestive system.

SERVES 4

SLOW COOKER
FREEZER-FRIENDLY

Prep time: 15 minutes

Cook time: 3 hours on high or 8 hours on low

2 (15-ounce) cans low-sodium cannellini beans, drained and rinsed

1½ cups frozen peas

3 carrots, peeled and diced

3 garlic cloves, minced

2 cups low-sodium vegetable broth

1 (28-ounce) can diced tomatoes

½ teaspoon salt

¼ teaspoon freshly ground black pepper

1. In a slow cooker, add the beans, peas, carrots, garlic, broth, tomatoes, salt, and pepper. Stir well to combine.

2. Cook on high for 3 hours or on low for 8 hours.

3. Serve warm or freeze for later. To freeze, store cooled chili in individual containers or one large freezer-safe container for up to 2 months. Defrost in the refrigerator overnight. Reheat in the microwave on high for several minutes depending on the portion size, or reheat in a pot over medium-low heat for 10 to 15 minutes.

TOBY'S TIP: Like a thicker stew? Whisk 1 tablespoon cornstarch with ¼ cup cool water, and stir it into the slow cooker 30 minutes before it's done cooking.

Serving size: 2 cups
Per serving: Calories: 277; Total fat: 2g; Saturated fat: 0g; Protein: 15g; Carbohydrates: 52g; Fiber: 16g; Sodium: 914mg

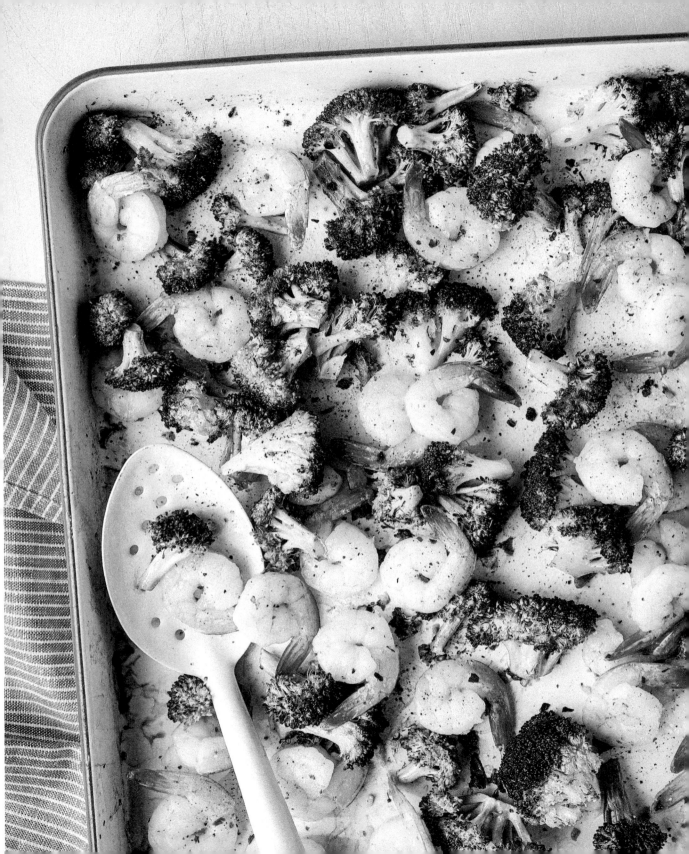

7 Fish and Seafood Mains

Mussels in Red Curry

GLUTEN-FREE | DAIRY-FREE | PALEO-FRIENDLY

I've always been intimidated by cooking shellfish, but I was pleasantly surprised by how easy it really is. The most important thing is to get your shellfish from a reputable market. Once you purchase it, keep it refrigerated and cook it within 24 hours.

SERVES 4

30-MINUTE

Prep time: 10 minutes

Cook time: 20 minutes

3 pounds mussels, scrubbed and debearded

2 cups low-sodium fish broth or chicken broth

1 tablespoon olive oil

1 garlic clove, minced

1 tablespoon red curry paste

1. Preheat the oven to 500°F.

2. Spread the mussels in a large baking dish.

3. Pour the broth over the mussels, and cover with aluminum foil.

4. Bake for 10 minutes, until the mussels open. Remove the foil and transfer the mussels to a large bowl, reserving the juices and discarding any that didn't open.

5. In a small saucepan over medium heat, heat the olive oil. Add the garlic and cook until fragrant, 1 minute. Add the reserved cooking juices and the curry paste, increase heat, and bring the mixture to a boil. Reduce heat and simmer for 5 minutes, until the flavors combine.

6. Divide the mussels evenly between 4 large bowls, and pour ½ cup of broth into each bowl.

TOBY'S TIP: Swap the mussels for clams, or use a combination of both. Whichever you choose to use, always toss those that have open shells before they've been cooked and those that don't open after cooking (it means they're dead and no good).

Serving size: 15 to 18 mussels plus ½ cup broth

Per serving: Calories: 351; Total fat: 13g; Saturated fat: 3g; Protein: 42g; Carbohydrates: 14g; Fiber: 0g; Sodium: 844mg

Sheet Pan Asian Shrimp with Broccoli

Shrimp has a reputation for being high in cholesterol, so some folks tend to shy away from it. However, the latest 2015–2020 Dietary Guidelines for Americans reviewed the scientific data and found that cholesterol in foods like shrimp and eggs don't raise blood cholesterol; rather, it's saturated fat that is responsible—and shrimp has very little. Now you can enjoy your shrimp without any guilt.

SERVES 4

FREEZER-FRIENDLY

Prep time: 15 minutes

Cook time: 20 minutes

Cooking spray

4 tablespoons olive oil, divided

2 garlic cloves, minced

1 teaspoon Italian seasoning

½ teaspoon salt, divided

¼ teaspoon freshly ground black pepper, divided

1 pound broccoli, cut into bite-size florets

⅛ teaspoon red pepper flakes

1½ pounds large shrimp, peeled, deveined, and tails removed

1. Preheat the oven to 400°F. Coat a large baking sheet with cooking spray.

2. In a medium bowl, whisk together 2 tablespoons of olive oil, the garlic, the Italian seasoning, ¼ teaspoon of salt, and ⅛ teaspoon of pepper.

3. Add the broccoli to the Italian seasoning mixture, and toss to coat.

4. Spread the broccoli in a single layer on the prepared baking sheet, and roast for 8 minutes.

5. Meanwhile, in the same medium bowl used for the broccoli, whisk together the remaining 2 tablespoons of olive oil, remaining ¼ teaspoon of salt, remaining ⅛ teaspoon of pepper, and the red pepper flakes. Add the shrimp and toss to coat.

6. Remove the pan from the oven, and add the shrimp to the broccoli, spreading in a single layer. Return the baking sheet to the oven and cook for an additional 10 minutes, until the shrimp are opaque and reach an internal cooking temperature of 145°F.

CONTINUED

Sheet Pan Asian Shrimp with Broccoli *continued*

7. Serve immediately or freeze for later. To freeze, place cooled shrimp and broccoli into a freezer-safe container in the freezer for up to 2 months. To defrost, refrigerate overnight. Reheat small batches in the microwave on high for about 2 minutes, or bake in a 350°F oven for about 10 minutes.

TOBY'S TIP: Serve this dish over soba noodles, rice noodles, or brown rice for a well-balanced meal.

Serving size: About 1 cup
Per serving: Calories: 274; Total fat: 15g; Saturated fat: 2g; Protein: 32g; Carbohydrates: 7g; Fiber: 0g; Sodium: 494mg

Creole Shrimp and Grits

GLUTEN-FREE | DAIRY-FREE

A traditional bowl of shrimp and grits can set you back hundreds of calories, especially with all the butter, sausage, and cheese. Luckily, you can whip up a mighty tasty version of this Southern-inspired treat with a fraction of the ingredients and calories.

SERVES 4

30-MINUTE

Prep time: 10 minutes

Cook time: 20 minutes

2¼ cups water, divided

½ cup quick-cooking grits or polenta

¼ teaspoon salt, divided

1 tablespoon olive oil

1½ pounds large shrimp, peeled and deveined

3 garlic cloves, minced

2 cups low-sodium chicken broth

1 teaspoon Creole seasoning

2 tablespoons cornstarch

⅛ teaspoon freshly ground black pepper

1 lemon, sliced

1. In a small saucepan, bring 2 cups of water to a boil. Stir the water while adding the grits and ⅛ teaspoon of salt. Reduce heat to low and simmer, covered, for about 7 minutes or until cooked through. Set aside to slightly cool.

2. In a large skillet over medium heat, heat the olive oil. Add the shrimp and cook until opaque, 2 minutes on each side. Using a slotted spoon, remove the shrimp from the skillet and transfer to a separate plate.

3. Add the garlic to the skillet and cook until fragrant, about 1 minute. Add the broth and Creole seasoning, and bring to a boil.

4. In a small bowl, mix the cornstarch with the remaining ¼ cup of water. Add the cornstarch mixture to the skillet and cook, stirring constantly, until the sauce thickens, about 2 minutes.

5. Return the shrimp to the skillet and cook, stirring occasionally, for 4 minutes.

6. Sprinkle with the remaining ⅛ teaspoon salt and the pepper.

7. To serve, distribute the grits among 4 bowls. Top each with ¼ of the shrimp and several lemon slices.

TOBY'S TIP: This spicy dish tastes even better with a dash hot sauce.

Serving size: ⅓ cup grits plus ¾ cup shrimp

Per serving: Calories: 224; Total fat: 4g; Saturated fat: 1g; Protein: 36g; Carbohydrates: 11g; Fiber: 1g; Sodium: 966mg

Soba Noodles with Cucumber, Avocado, and Crab

DAIRY-FREE

Order a noodle dish at an Asian restaurant and you'll probably find it glistening in oil and packed with close to 1,000 calories. Instead, you can whip up a quick and easy soba noodle dish in minutes with a fraction of the calories.

SERVES 4

30-MINUTE

Prep time: 15 minutes

Cook time: 10 minutes

8 ounces soba (buckwheat) noodles

1 large cucumber, diced

1 ripe avocado, pitted, peeled, and diced

1 pound canned crabmeat, drained and gently rinsed

¼ cup Thai Dressing (page 183)

1. Fill a large pot with water and bring to a boil over high heat. Add the soba noodles and cook until tender, about 8 minutes. Drain in a colander and rinse under cold water. Transfer the noodles to a large bowl and set aside to cool.

2. Once cooled, add the cucumber, avocado, and crabmeat, and toss to combine.

3. Drizzle the Thai Dressing over the noodles, and gently toss to evenly coat.

TOBY'S TIP: The cooking time of soba noodles varies. Check the package for specific cooking times.

Serving size: About 2 cups
Per serving: Calories: 476; Total fat: 22g; Saturated fat: 3g; Protein: 24g; Carbohydrates: 51g; Fiber: 7g; Sodium: 658mg

Greek-Style Fish Pitas

Growing up in a home surrounded by Israeli foods, I learned to stuff pita with almost anything. My basic go-tos are chopped salad and tahini or hummus, but I'll always switch up the protein from lamb to fish to falafel to chicken. This recipe employs a light, flaky tilapia.

SERVES 4

30-MINUTE

Prep time: 15 minutes

Cook time: 15 minutes

1 pound tilapia

1 teaspoon dried oregano

¼ teaspoon salt

⅛ teaspoon freshly ground black pepper

2 tablespoons olive oil

Juice of 1 lemon

4 (6½-inch) whole-wheat pitas, cut open at the top

¼ cup Tahini Yogurt Sauce (page 186) or store-bought hummus

1 cup Mediterranean Chopped Salad (page 41)

1. Preheat the oven to 350°F.

2. Sprinkle both sides of the tilapia with the oregano, salt, and pepper.

3. In a medium skillet over medium heat, heat the olive oil. Add the tilapia and cook for 8 minutes, flipping once halfway through, until the fish is opaque and has reached an internal temperature of 145°F. Add the lemon juice, evenly coating the fish.

4. Remove from heat and allow the fish to slightly cool before cutting it into about 8 equal pieces.

5. On two baking sheets, distribute the pitas in a single layer. Warm in the oven for about 5 minutes. Remove from the oven and allow to slightly cool.

6. Use clean fingers to pry a pita open at the top. Add 2 pieces of fish, 1 tablespoon sauce or hummus, and ¼ cup salad. Repeat with the remaining pitas.

TOBY'S TIP: To make these stuffed pitas dairy-free, opt for hummus instead of the Tahini Yogurt Sauce. Or make them vegetarian by switching out the fish for Baked Lentil Falafel (page 86).

Serving size: 1 fish pita
Per serving: Calories: 392; Total fat: 14g; Saturated fat: 2g; Protein: 32g; Carbohydrates: 39g; Fiber: 6g; Sodium: 634mg

Simple Fish Stew

When the cold weather settles in, my body craves warming dishes, like stews. In particular, the combination of a warm tomato base with bite-size pieces of fish, beef, or beans creates a cozy feeling and keeps me satisfied. This stew can also be made with another firm fish, like halibut or sea bass.

SERVES 4

30-MINUTE

Prep time: 5 minutes

Cook time: 25 minutes

2 (14-ounce cans) no-added-sodium diced tomatoes, divided

2 tablespoons olive oil

1 onion, diced

3 garlic cloves, minced

2 tablespoons herbes de Provence

1 (8-ounce) bottle clam juice

1¼ pounds cod, cut into 2-inch chunks

¼ teaspoon salt

⅛ teaspoon freshly ground black pepper

1. Pour 1 can of diced tomatoes into a blender. Blend until smooth.

2. In a large saucepan over medium heat, heat the olive oil. Add the onion and cook until soft and translucent, 3 minutes. Add the garlic and herbes de Provence, and cook until fragrant, 1 minute.

3. Add the blended tomatoes, the remaining can of diced tomatoes, and the clam juice. Bring the mixture to a boil, then reduce heat and simmer for 10 minutes, until the flavors combine.

4. Add the cod, cover, and poach for about 10 minutes, until cooked through and the internal temperature of the fish reaches 145°F.

5. Season with the salt and pepper, and stir to combine.

TOBY'S TIP: Herbes de Provence is one of the most popular spice blends. It's made from a combination of herbs—usually thyme, marjoram, rosemary, oregano, and savory. Sprinkle on baked fries or Easy Sautéed Chicken Breast (page 118), or use it in Herbed Pork Meatballs (page 148) if you can't get your hands on fresh herbs.

Serving size: 1¾ cups
Per serving: Calories: 218; Total fat: 7g; Saturated fat: 1g; Protein: 24g; Carbohydrates: 13g; Fiber: 2g; Sodium: 881mg

Braised Cod over Tomatoes

Any dish that takes 30 minutes or less is a winner in my book. If you slice the tomatoes in the morning before heading to work, you can shave off about 5 minutes and have a delicious 200-calorie dinner ready in 20 minutes flat.

SERVES 4

**ONE POT/ONE PAN
30-MINUTE**

Prep time: 10 minutes

Cook time: 15 minutes

1¼ pounds cod, cut into 4 equal pieces

¼ teaspoon salt

⅛ teaspoon freshly ground black pepper

2 tablespoons olive oil

2 pounds (about 8) Roma or plum tomatoes, cut into ¼-inch-thick slices

1 garlic clove, sliced

1 tablespoon dried oregano

⅛ teaspoon red pepper flakes

Juice of ½ lemon

1. Sprinkle both sides of the cod with the salt and pepper.

2. In a large skillet over medium heat, heat the olive oil. When the oil is shimmering, layer the tomatoes evenly on the bottom of the skillet. Sprinkle with the garlic, oregano, and red pepper flakes. Place the cod evenly over the tomatoes. Cover and cook for about 15 minutes, until the fish is opaque and reaches an internal temperature of 145°F.

3. Transfer the fish to a serving dish, leaving the tomatoes in the skillet. Break up the tomatoes with the back of a spoon, and drizzle them with the lemon juice.

4. Spoon the tomatoes over the fish and serve.

TOBY'S TIP: For a spin on this dish, swap the tomatoes for leeks or a combination of fennel and tomatoes.

Serving size: 1 piece cod plus ¼ of the tomatoes

Per serving: Calories: 204; Total fat: 8g; Saturated fat: 1g; Protein: 24g; Carbohydrates: 10g; Fiber: 3g; Sodium: 589mg

Oven-Steamed Halibut with Carrots, Tomatoes, and Thyme

Halibut is one of the lower-fat fish options available. A 3-ounce serving has 115 calories, 2.5 grams of fat, and 22 grams of protein. Its flaky consistency and ability to hold together during cooking make halibut a healthy, delicious fish option for a variety of dishes.

SERVES 4

ONE POT/ONE PAN
30-MINUTE

Prep time: 10 minutes

Cook time: 20 minutes

4 (5-ounce) skin-on halibut fillets

½ teaspoon salt, divided

1 tablespoon olive oil

1 onion, chopped

2 garlic cloves, minced

2 medium carrots, peeled into ribbons

1 cup cherry tomatoes, halved

4 thyme sprigs

⅛ teaspoon freshly ground black pepper

1. Preheat the oven to 400°F.

2. Sprinkle the flesh side of the fish with ¼ teaspoon of salt.

3. In an ovenproof pan over medium heat, heat the olive oil. When the oil is shimmering, add the onion and cook until translucent, about 3 minutes. Add the garlic and cook until fragrant, an additional 1 minute.

4. Scatter the carrots and tomatoes evenly around the pan, and top with the halibut, skin-side down, and the thyme. Sprinkle with the remaining ¼ teaspoon of salt and the pepper. Cover the pan with a lid or aluminum foil, and bake for about 15 minutes, until the fish is opaque and reaches an internal temperature of 145°F.

5. Remove from the oven and allow to cool for 10 minutes. Serve warm.

TOBY'S TIP: Substitute the halibut with another white fish, like flounder or cod.

Serving size: 1 halibut fillet plus ⅓ cup vegetables
Per serving: Calories: 192; Total fat: 5g; Saturated fat: 1g; Protein: 27g; Carbohydrates: 8g; Fiber: 2g; Sodium: 415mg

Sea Bass with Rustic Tomato and Fennel Sauce

GLUTEN-FREE | DAIRY-FREE | PALEO-FRIENDLY

Fennel pairs beautifully with sea bass in this savory dish. One cup of this licorice-tasting veggie provides 27 calories and 3 grams of fiber. It's a good source of vitamin C, potassium, and folate. Fennel also contains a phytochemical (natural plant chemical) called anethole, which has been shown to help reduce inflammation and aid with digestion, and may also help prevent cancer.

SERVES 4

ONE POT/ONE PAN

Prep time: 15 minutes

Cook time: 20 minutes

Cooking spray

1 medium fennel bulb

1 red onion, thinly sliced

4 plum tomatoes, diced

2 lemons

4 (5-ounce) sea bass fillets

¼ teaspoon salt

⅛ teaspoon freshly ground black pepper

2 tablespoons olive oil

1 teaspoon mustard

1 garlic clove, minced

1. Preheat the oven to 450°F. Coat a baking sheet with cooking spray.

2. Remove the fronds from the fennel bulb and set aside. Finely chop the fennel bulb and the fronds separately.

3. Evenly scatter the fennel bulb, onion, and tomatoes on the prepared baking sheet.

4. Bake for 5 minutes, until the vegetables soften.

5. Meanwhile, cut 1 lemon into thin slices. Sprinkle the sea bass with the salt and pepper.

6. Remove the baking sheet from the oven, and top the vegetables with the fish. Place the lemon slices over the fish. Return to the oven and bake for 15 minutes, until the fish is opaque and reaches an internal temperature of 145°F.

7. Meanwhile, juice the second lemon. In a small bowl, whisk together the lemon juice, olive oil, mustard, garlic, and chopped fennel fronds to make a dressing.

8. To serve, place 1 sea bass fillet on each of 4 plates, and top each with ¾ cup of vegetables and 1 tablespoon of dressing.

TOBY'S TIP: Swap the tomatoes for mandarin oranges, pears, or grapefruit. All will help mellow the licorice taste of the fennel.

Serving size: 1 sea bass fillet plus ¾ cup vegetables and 1 tablespoon dressing
Per serving: Calories: 240; Total fat: 10g; Saturated fat: 2g; Protein: 28g; Carbohydrates: 10g; Fiber: 3g; Sodium: 293mg

Spiced Tilapia with Mango Chutney

GLUTEN-FREE | DAIRY-FREE

This is a great summertime dish. Mango, a cousin of the cashew and pistachio (yes, really!), was brought to Miami in 1862 from the West Indies. Mangos are packed with nutrition, with 1 cup providing 107 calories, 28 grams of carbs, and 3 grams of fiber, and they contain over 20 vitamins and minerals. This gorgeously hued fruit also contains natural compounds called flavonoids, which may help control high blood pressure and reduce the risk of stroke and heart disease.

SERVES 4

ONE POT/ONE PAN
30-MINUTE

Prep time: 10 minutes

Cook time: 10 minutes

Cooking spray

1¼ pounds tilapia,
cut into 4 fillets

2 tablespoons olive oil

½ teaspoon garlic powder

½ teaspoon paprika

½ teaspoon Italian seasoning

¼ teaspoon salt

⅛ teaspoon freshly ground
black pepper

½ cup Easy Mango
Chutney (page 191)

1. Preheat the broiler. Coat a baking sheet with cooking spray.

2. Brush both sides of the tilapia with the olive oil.

3. In a small bowl, mix together the garlic powder, paprika, Italian seasoning, salt, and pepper.

4. Sprinkle both sides of the tilapia with the spice mixture, and place in a single layer on the prepared baking sheet. Broil for 5 minutes on each side, until the fish is flaky and reaches an internal cooking temperature of 145°F.

5. Place one tilapia fillet on each of 4 plates, and top each with 2 tablespoons of chutney.

TOBY'S TIP: To save time during the busy workweek, whip up a batch of Easy Mango Chutney (page 191) up to 3 days in advance.

Serving size: 1 tilapia fillet plus 2 tablespoons chutney
Per serving: Calories: 231; Total fat: 9g; Saturated fat: 2g; Protein: 29g; Carbohydrates: 9g; Fiber: 1g; Sodium: 223mg

Pistachio-Crusted Flounder

GLUTEN-FREE | DAIRY-FREE

Besides having a delicious flavor and fabulous crunch, pistachios bring lots of reasons to love them. According to the U.S. Department of Agriculture Nutrient Database, pistachios provide more than 30 different vitamins, minerals, and phytonutrients. One ounce of pistachios (49 nuts) contains 160 calories and 6 grams of protein. Further, the Food and Drug Administration has found that eating 1½ ounces of most nuts per day, as part of a diet low in saturated fat and cholesterol, may help reduce the risk of heart disease.

SERVES 4

30-MINUTE

Prep time: 15 minutes

Cook time: 15 minutes

Cooking spray

¼ cup gluten-free Dijon mustard

½ teaspoon salt, divided

⅛ teaspoon freshly ground black pepper

½ cup raw shelled pistachios, finely chopped

2 tablespoons cornmeal

¼ cup chopped fresh parsley

4 (5-ounce) flounder fillets

1. Preheat the oven to 400°F. Coat a baking sheet with cooking spray.

2. In a small bowl, whisk together the Dijon mustard, ¼ teaspoon of salt, and the pepper. Set aside.

3. In another small bowl, mix together the pistachios, cornmeal, parsley, and remaining ¼ teaspoon of salt.

4. Brush both sides of 1 flounder fillet with the mustard mixture, and then dredge both sides in the pistachio mixture, pressing down with clean fingers to make sure the pistachios stick. Place the flounder on the prepared baking sheet. Repeat with the remaining 3 fillets, leaving ½ inch between pieces.

5. Bake for about 15 minutes, until the fish is cooked through and reaches an internal temperature of 145°F.

TOBY'S TIP: Swap the pistachios for pecans or almonds—whatever you have lying around.

Serving size: 1 flounder fillet
Per serving: Calories: 243; Total fat: 9g; Saturated fat: 1g; Protein: 30g; Carbohydrates: 10g; Fiber: 2g; Sodium: 573mg

Mediterranean Trout in Parchment Paper

When cooking fish, meat, veggies, or herbs in parchment paper, you're steaming the ingredients inside using their own moisture. Unless you add oil or butter for flavor, there is no fat required. The best part? There's no need to pile up dirty dishes, so the only cleanup is walking to the trash and tossing the paper!

SERVES 4

ONE POT/ONE PAN
30-MINUTE

Prep time: 15 minutes
Cook time: 10 minutes

4 (5-ounce) skin-on trout or grouper fillets

½ teaspoon salt, divided

¼ teaspoon freshly ground black pepper, divided

2 tablespoons olive oil

2 tablespoons white cooking wine

1 garlic clove, minced

1 cup cherry tomatoes, halved lengthwise

1 red onion, thinly sliced

¼ cup Kalamata olives, halved lengthwise

1 lemon, sliced

1. Preheat the oven to 400°F.

2. Sprinkle the flesh side of the fish with ¼ teaspoon of salt and ⅛ teaspoon of pepper.

3. In a small bowl, whisk together the olive oil, wine, garlic, remaining ¼ teaspoon of salt, and remaining ⅛ teaspoon of pepper.

4. Place a piece of parchment paper flat on the counter. On the lower half, place 1 trout fillet and top with ¼ each of the cherry tomatoes, onion, olives, and lemon slices. Fold the parchment paper in half over the fish. Working your way around, gently roll the edges of the open sides of the paper, tucking the ends under the packet. Repeat this step for the remaining 3 fillets.

5. Place 2 packets on each of 2 baking sheets, and bake for 10 minutes, until the fish is opaque and reaches an internal temperature of 145°F. Using a sharp knife, carefully cut several 3-inch slits in the packets to let steam escape. Serve warm.

TOBY'S TIP: You can buy parchment paper bags made for cooking fish *en papillote*, the French term for "in parchment." You can also use aluminum foil to cook the fish in this manner.

Serving size: 1 packet
Per serving: Calories: 320; Total fat: 18g; Saturated fat: 3g; Protein: 30g; Carbohydrates: 6g; Fiber: 1g; Sodium: 572mg

Coconut Curry Salmon

I try to include fatty fish, like salmon and tuna, in my diet several times a week. These fish are packed with omega-3 fats, specifically one called DHA. Your brain needs omega-3s throughout your life, especially DHA, which is most abundant in your brain. However, the DHA must be replenished regularly. Research shows that DHA contributes to improved memory function in older adults and is also important for the brain development of babies.

SERVES 4

ONE POT/ONE PAN
30-MINUTE

Prep time: 5 minutes

Cook time: 15 minutes

½ cup unsweetened coconut flakes

2 tablespoons olive oil

1¼ pounds skin-on salmon

Zest and juice of 2 limes

¼ cup water

½ cup coconut milk

¼ teaspoon curry powder

½ teaspoon salt

1. In a medium sauté pan or skillet over medium heat, toast the coconut for 3 minutes, until browned. Set aside to slightly cool.

2. Using a clean paper towel, wipe out the pan, then add the olive oil and heat over medium heat. When the oil is shimmering, add the salmon, skin-side down, and sprinkle with the lime zest. Add the water, cover, and steam for 8 to 10 minutes, until cooked through with an internal temperature of 145°F.

3. Transfer the salmon to a serving platter. Return the pan to medium heat, and cook off any extra liquid in the pan.

4. Add the lime juice, coconut milk, toasted coconut flakes, curry powder, and salt, and bring to a boil. Reduce heat to a simmer and cook for 2 minutes, stirring occasionally.

5. Cut the fish into 4 equal pieces. Spoon the sauce over the fish and serve warm.

TOBY'S TIP: For small amounts of flavorful foods, like the coconut milk in this recipe, I opt for the full-fat variety. It lends to the creaminess and flavor of the sauce without weighing the recipe down with calories.

Serving size: 1 piece salmon plus 2 tablespoons sauce
Per serving: Calories: 366; Total fat: 26g; Saturated fat: 12g; Protein: 29g; Carbohydrates: 4g; Fiber: 1g; Sodium: 221mg

Slow Cooker Salmon with Leeks and Asparagus

GLUTEN-FREE | DAIRY-FREE | PALEO-FRIENDLY

Once I bought a slow cooker and mastered chili and pork loin, I was on a mission to create all kinds of foods with my prized kitchen equipment. Recently, I moved into cooking salmon with vegetables. I pop the salmon and vegetables of my choice with vegetable broth or a combo of wine and water, and let it cook on low for about 2 hours. By dinnertime, I've got a restaurant-style meal ready to go, and now you can, too.

SERVES 4

SLOW COOKER

Prep time: 15 minutes

Cook time: 2 to 2½ hours

1¼ pounds skin-on salmon

¼ teaspoon salt

⅛ teaspoon freshly ground black pepper

1 leek, cleaned and chopped

¾ pound asparagus, trimmed and halved crosswise

¾ cup water

¾ cup white cooking wine

1. Cut a large piece of aluminum foil or parchment paper and line the bottom of the slow cooker.

2. Sprinkle the flesh side of the salmon with the salt and pepper.

3. Place the salmon skin-side down in the bottom of the slow cooker. Top the salmon with the leek, asparagus, water, and wine. Cook on low for 2 to 2½ hours.

4. Lift out the foil or parchment paper, and gently slide the salmon and vegetables onto a serving plate. Serve warm.

TOBY'S TIP: Once cooked, remove the salmon and vegetables from the slow cooker immediately; otherwise the vegetables will oversoften.

Serving size: 5 ounces salmon plus ¼ of the vegetables

Per serving: Calories: 236; Total fat: 9g; Saturated fat: 1g; Protein: 30g; Carbohydrates: 7g; Fiber: 2g; Sodium: 217mg

Miso-Glazed Tuna

GLUTEN-FREE | DAIRY-FREE

After college, I rented an apartment in New York City and started to learn how to cook all kinds of dishes. Tuna was the first fish I learned how to prepare. I would marinate it with a teriyaki sauce and grill it on my George Foreman Grill, which everyone had in the 1990s. I've swapped my George Foreman Grill for a grill pan, but now I opt to cook tuna using different cooking methods, including in the oven.

SERVES 4

FREEZER-FRIENDLY

Prep time: 10 minutes,
plus 30 minutes to chill
Cook time: 15 minutes

Cooking spray

⅓ cup white miso

⅓ cup sake

⅓ cup mirin

2 tablespoons brown sugar

4 (5-ounce) tuna steaks

1. Preheat the oven to 400°F. Coat an ovenproof baking dish with cooking spray.

2. In a small saucepan over low heat, whisk together the miso, sake, mirin, and brown sugar. Whisk continuously until the sugar is melted, about 2 minutes.

3. Pour the glaze into a medium bowl. Add the tuna, turning to coat. Cover and place in the refrigerator for at least 30 minutes but no longer than overnight.

4. Remove the tuna from the glaze and place in the prepared baking dish. Discard any remaining glaze. Bake for 12 minutes, or until the fish is opaque and cooked to a minimum internal temperature of 145°F.

5. Serve the fish warm or freeze for later. To freeze, place cooled fish into a freezer-safe container and freeze for up to 2 months. To defrost, refrigerate overnight. Reheat one piece at a time in the microwave on high for 1½ minutes, or in a 350°F oven for about 10 minutes.

TOBY'S TIP: Round out your meal by adding veggies to your Asian-inspired tuna! Add 2 cups snow peas and 8 ounces sliced shiitake mushrooms in the baking dish with the tuna steaks. Also, in a pinch, you can use rice wine instead of mirin and sake, though sake is sweeter.

Serving size: 1 tuna steak
Per serving: Calories: 271; Total fat: 1g; Saturated fat: 0g; Protein: 37g; Carbohydrates: 23g; Fiber: 2g; Sodium: 959mg

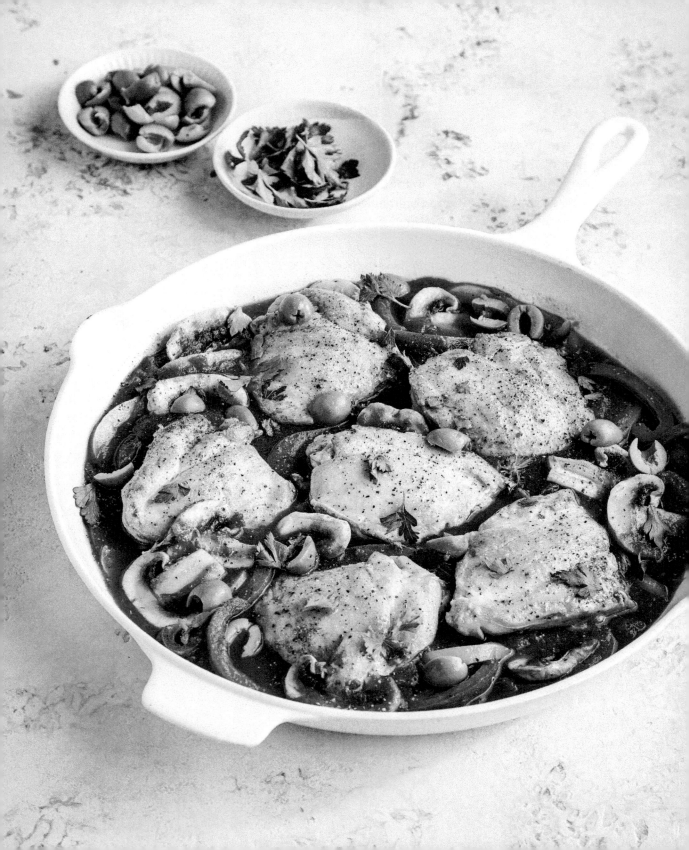

8

Chicken and Turkey Mains

Easy Sautéed Chicken Breast

GLUTEN-FREE | DAIRY-FREE | PALEO-FRIENDLY

When I teach folks how to cook, one of the first recipes I suggest learning is sautéed chicken breast on the stovetop. Once you master that recipe, you can use the same simple flavors and grill the chicken breasts on an outdoor grill or grill pan. It takes small steps to be able to walk, but after a while you'll be running around creating all sorts of chicken dishes.

SERVES 4

ONE POT/ONE PAN
FREEZER-FRIENDLY

Prep time: 15 minutes

Cook time: 20 minutes

4 (5-ounce) skinless, boneless chicken breasts

¼ teaspoon salt

⅛ teaspoon freshly ground black pepper

2 tablespoons olive oil

Juice of 1 lemon

1. Loosely wrap each chicken breast in plastic wrap and place on a cutting board. Using a mallet or heavy-bottomed pan, pound the chicken until each breast is about 1 inch thick. Unwrap the chicken, and discard the plastic wrap.

2. Season the chicken on both sides with the salt and pepper.

3. In a large skillet over medium heat, heat the olive oil. When the oil is shimmering, add the chicken breasts and cook on one side until browned, about 10 minutes. Flip the chicken over and drizzle with the lemon juice. Continue cooking for about 10 minutes, until the chicken is cooked through and the internal temperature reaches 165°F.

4. Serve immediately or freeze for later. To freeze, store cooled chicken in a freezer-safe container in the freezer for up to 2 months. To defrost, refrigerate overnight. Reheat one breast at a time in the microwave on high for 1 minute.

TOBY'S TIP: Use these sautéed chicken breasts for the Leftover Chicken Soup (page 39), Brussels Sprout Caesar Salad with Chicken (page 48), Chicken Nacho Bites (page 80), or Pesto Pasta with Chicken (page 120).

Serving size: 1 chicken breast
Per serving: Calories: 232; Total fat: 10g; Saturated fat: 2g; Protein: 32g; Carbohydrates: 1g; Fiber: 0g; Sodium: 211mg

Chicken Quesadillas

If you love to order quesadillas when you're out to eat, you can expect to rack up close to 1,000 calories. Oftentimes they're overloaded with cheese and come with high-calorie dips, like sour cream and guac. This lighter version uses flavorful chicken and just enough cheese, and provides a spicy jalapeño kick for a meal that comes in under 500 calories per serving.

SERVES 4

30-MINUTE

Prep time: 10 minutes

Cook time: 10 minutes

Cooking spray

1 tablespoon olive oil

1 pound Easy Sautéed Chicken Breast (page 118) or leftover chicken, cut into bite-size pieces

1½ teaspoons ground cumin

¼ teaspoon salt

⅛ teaspoon freshly ground black pepper

8 (8-inch) whole-wheat tortillas

1 jalapeño pepper, seeded and thinly sliced

1½ cups low-fat shredded Monterey Jack cheese

1. Preheat the oven to 400°F. Coat two baking sheets with cooking spray.

2. In a medium skillet over medium heat, heat the olive oil. Add the chicken pieces and warm through, about 2 minutes. Add the cumin, salt, and pepper, tossing to evenly coat.

3. Coat one side of 4 tortillas with cooking spray, and place 2 tortillas coated-side down on each baking sheet. Divide the chicken evenly between the 4 tortillas, and use the back of a spoon to spread the chicken to the edge of the tortillas. Sprinkle each tortilla with 3 or 4 jalapeño slices and ⅓ cup of cheese, and top with a tortilla. Use clean hands to gently press down on the quesadilla.

4. Bake for 8 minutes, until cheese has melted and tortillas are slightly browned.

5. Remove from the oven and allow to cool for 5 minutes. Slice each quesadilla into 4 quarters.

TOBY'S TIP: Serve with Simple Salsa (page 189) and nonfat plain Greek yogurt.

Serving size: 1 quesadilla

Per serving: Calories: 606; Total fat: 29g; Saturated fat: 12g; Protein: 46g; Carbohydrates: 39g; Fiber: 8g; Sodium: 977mg

Pesto Pasta with Chicken

This book shows that you don't have to slave over a hot stove to get a quick and easy well-balanced dinner on the table, and this recipe is a great example. Oftentimes, leftovers in the refrigerator can be tossed together to make a delicious meal like this one. Pesto pasta is a go-to in my world, but I add chicken to ensure I stay feeling full well after dinner is over.

SERVES 4

30-MINUTE

Prep time: 15 minutes

Cook time: 15 minutes

12 ounces whole-grain spaghetti

8 ounces Easy Sautéed Chicken Breast (page 118) or leftover chicken, cut into bite-size pieces

¾ cup Easy Pesto Sauce (page 185) or store-bought pesto

1 cup cherry tomatoes, halved

¼ teaspoon salt

⅛ teaspoon freshly ground black pepper

¼ cup grated Parmesan cheese

1. Fill a large pot with water and bring to a boil over high heat. Add the spaghetti and cook, stirring often, until al dente, about 9 minutes. Drain the spaghetti and place in a large skillet.

2. Add the chicken to the skillet and toss with the spaghetti over medium-low heat to warm the chicken. Add the pesto, tossing to evenly coat. Add the tomatoes, salt, and pepper, and continue cooking for about 5 minutes, until the flavors combine.

3. Transfer the pasta to a large serving bowl, and sprinkle with the Parmesan cheese.

TOBY'S TIP: To make this dish gluten-free, opt for pasta made from quinoa, chickpeas, or lentils. Try a few varieties to figure out your favorites.

Serving size: 2 cups
Per serving: Calories: 548; Total fat: 21g; Saturated fat: 4g; Protein: 28g; Carbohydrates: 67g; Fiber: 1g; Sodium: 633mg

Sweet and Spicy Chicken Fingers

GLUTEN-FREE | DAIRY-FREE

You can make healthy and delectable chicken fingers with five ingredients, and without frying! This quick and easy baked version uses honey and brown rice cereal, plus a little spice from sriracha. Enjoy these for dinner or serve as an appetizer for your game-day spread.

SERVES 4

Prep time: 20 minutes

Cook time: 30 minutes

Cooking spray

1¼ pounds skinless, boneless chicken breast tenders

¼ teaspoon salt

⅛ teaspoon freshly ground black pepper

3 cups brown rice cereal

½ cup honey

2 teaspoons sriracha

1. Preheat the oven to 375°F. Coat a baking sheet with cooking spray.

2. Sprinkle both sides of the chicken with salt and pepper.

3. Place the brown rice cereal in a resealable plastic bag. Using a rolling pin, crush the cereal into small pieces, then pour into a large bowl.

4. In a medium bowl, whisk together the honey and sriracha.

5. Dip each chicken tender in the honey mixture, allowing the excess to drip off. Then dredge in the rice cereal, pressing to evenly coat both sides. Place the chicken tenders on the prepared baking sheet, leaving about ½ inch of space between them. Bake for 30 minutes, until the chicken is browned and reaches an internal temperature of 165°F.

TOBY'S TIP: Serve these chicken fingers with Homemade Honey Mustard (page 181).

Serving size: 2 or 3 chicken fingers

Per serving: Calories: 331; Total fat: 4g; Saturated fat: 1g; Protein: 33g; Carbohydrates: 41g; Fiber: 1g; Sodium: 320mg

Cilantro-Lime Chicken

GLUTEN-FREE | DAIRY-FREE | PALEO-FRIENDLY

Cilantro complements citrus fruits, like lime, beautifully. Plus, this herb is packed with folate and vitamins A, C, and K. Though a small amount won't do very much, using cilantro regularly in dishes provides fresh flavor while allowing the nutrients to add up.

SERVES 4

FREEZER-FRIENDLY

Prep time: 15 minutes, plus 30 minutes to chill
Cook time: 30 minutes

3 limes

⅓ cup chopped cilantro

2 garlic cloves, minced

1 tablespoon brown sugar

⅛ teaspoon red pepper flakes

¼ teaspoon salt

⅛ teaspoon freshly ground black pepper

1¼ pounds skinless, boneless chicken thighs

Cooking spray

2 tablespoons olive oil

1. Zest and juice 2 limes. Slice the third lime and set aside.

2. In a small bowl, whisk together the lime zest and juice, cilantro, garlic, brown sugar, red pepper flakes, salt, and pepper. Add the chicken and toss to combine. Cover the bowl and marinate in the refrigerator for at least 30 minutes and up to overnight.

3. Preheat the oven to 350°F. Coat an 8-by-8-inch ovenproof baking dish with cooking spray.

4. In a medium skillet over medium-high heat, heat the olive oil. Add the chicken thighs and the marinade, and bring the liquid to a boil. Reduce heat to medium and cook until the chicken is browned, about 5 minutes on each side.

5. Transfer the chicken and the sauce into the prepared baking dish. Place the lime slices on top of the chicken. Cover with aluminum foil and bake for about 20 minutes, until the chicken reaches an internal temperature of 165°F.

6. Serve immediately or freeze for later. To freeze, place cooled chicken in a resealable container in the freezer for up to 2 months. To defrost, refrigerate overnight. Reheat single portions in the microwave on high for 2 minutes, or bake in a 350°F oven for 15 to 20 minutes, until warmed through.

TOBY'S TIP: Although olive oil is used in most of the recipes in this book, including this one, you can always substitute canola or safflower oil. Both have a mild flavor and can withstand higher cooking temperatures.

Serving size: 5 ounces chicken
Per serving: Calories: 354; Total fat: 26g; Saturated fat: 7g; Protein: 24g; Carbohydrates: 6g; Fiber: 1g; Sodium: 264mg

Spanish-Style Chicken in Tomato Sauce

GLUTEN-FREE | DAIRY-FREE | PALEO-FRIENDLY

Chicken thighs may be dark meat, but they can still be part of your healthy eating plan. Dark meat is high in healthy monounsaturated fat, and it's usually more affordable than chicken breasts. Opt to purchase skinless dark meat or remove it yourself, as the skin is where most of the artery-clogging saturated fat is found.

SERVES 4

ONE POT/ONE PAN
FREEZER-FRIENDLY

Prep time: 15 minutes

Cook time: 40 minutes

1¼ pounds skinless, boneless chicken thighs

½ teaspoon salt, divided

¼ teaspoon freshly ground black pepper, divided

2 tablespoons olive oil, divided

1 onion, chopped

1 garlic clove, minced

2 green bell peppers, seeded and cut into ¼-inch strips

10 ounces white mushrooms, thinly sliced

1 (28-ounce) can crushed tomatoes

2 tablespoons chopped fresh parsley, for garnish (optional)

¼ cup halved and pitted green olives, for garnish (optional)

1. Season both sides of the chicken with ¼ teaspoon of salt and ⅛ teaspoon of pepper.

2. In a large skillet over medium heat, heat 1 tablespoon of olive oil. When the oil is shimmering, add the chicken and cook for 10 minutes, flipping once, until both sides are browned. Remove the chicken from the skillet and set aside.

3. In the skillet, heat the remaining 1 tablespoon of olive oil over medium heat. When the oil is shimmering, add the onion and cook until translucent, 3 minutes. Add the garlic and cook until fragrant, 1 minute. Add the peppers and mushrooms, and cook for 5 minutes, until the vegetables begin to soften.

4. Add the crushed tomatoes and bring the mixture to a boil. Return the chicken to the skillet and toss to coat. Reduce heat and simmer, covered, for 20 to 25 minutes, until the chicken is cooked through. Add the remaining ¼ teaspoon salt and remaining ⅛ teaspoon pepper, and stir to combine.

CONTINUED

5. Serve warm garnished with the parsley and olives, if desired, or freeze for later. To freeze, place cooled chicken with tomato sauce into a resealable container in the freezer for up to 2 months. To defrost, refrigerate overnight. Reheat in a large skillet over medium heat until heated through, about 12 minutes. Single-serve portions can be reheated in the microwave on high for 2 minutes.

TOBY'S TIP: Any color bell pepper works in this recipe. Swap out the green for red or yellow bell peppers, or use a combination. And for even more flavor, add ¼ cup olives and 2 tablespoons fresh parsley leaves to the dish.

Serving size: 1¾ cups
Per serving: Calories: 476; Total fat: 31g; Saturated fat: 8g; Protein: 30g; Carbohydrates: 23g; Fiber: 6g; Sodium: 785mg

Light and Simple Chicken Parmesan

One of my favorite dishes is chicken Parmesan, and it has become a favorite of my son's as well. However, most restaurants deep-fry the chicken and then coat it with tons of full-fat cheese. I know this recipe satisfies, because when my son smells this dish cooking, he comes running out of his room immediately—and he's a teenager who never leaves his room!

SERVES 4

FREEZER-FRIENDLY

Prep time: 15 minutes

Cook time: 30 minutes

Cooking spray

4 (5-ounce) skinless, boneless chicken breasts

2 cups Basic Tomato Sauce (page 184) or jarred tomato sauce, divided

1 cup Homemade Bread Crumbs (page 192) or store-bought unseasoned bread crumbs

½ cup grated Parmesan cheese, divided

¼ teaspoon salt

⅛ teaspoon freshly ground black pepper

1½ cups shredded part-skim mozzarella cheese

1. Preheat the oven to 350°F. Coat a 9-by-13-inch baking dish with cooking spray.

2. Loosely wrap each chicken breast in plastic wrap and place on a cutting board. Using a mallet or heavy-bottomed pan, pound the chicken until each breast is about 1 inch thick. Unwrap the chicken and discard the plastic wrap.

3. Spread 1 cup of tomato sauce onto the bottom of the prepared baking dish.

4. In a large bowl, combine the bread crumbs, ¼ cup of Parmesan cheese, and the salt and pepper.

5. Coat both sides of the chicken with cooking spray. Dredge both sides in the bread crumb mixture, pressing down so the bread crumbs stick to the chicken. Place the breaded chicken into the prepared baking dish.

6. Top the chicken with the remaining 1 cup of tomato sauce, and use the back of a large spoon to spread it evenly over the chicken. Sprinkle the mozzarella evenly over the chicken, and sprinkle with the remaining ¼ cup of Parmesan cheese.

CONTINUED

7. Cover the dish with aluminum foil and bake for 30 minutes, until bubbly with an internal temperature of 165°F.

8. Serve warm or freeze for later. To freeze, place into a resealable container in the freezer for up to 2 months. To defrost, refrigerate overnight. Reheat in an ovenproof dish at 350°F for 15 to 20 minutes, until warmed through. Reheat individual portions in the microwave on high for 2 to 2½ minutes.

TOBY'S TIP: Serve this dish with Spicy Roasted Broccoli with Garlic (page 56) or Sautéed Spinach with Shallots (page 58).

Serving size: 1 chicken breast plus ¼ of the sauce
Per serving: Calories: 413; Total fat: 16g; Saturated fat: 7g; Protein: 49g; Carbohydrates: 15g; Fiber: 2g; Sodium: 850mg

Chicken Marsala

DAIRY-FREE

Ordering chicken Marsala at a restaurant will set you back around 1,100 calories, and that's without the bread, starter salad, dessert, or glass of wine. Luckily, this lighter version, which lightly dredges the chicken in a touch of flour, keeps the calories in check at 414 per serving.

SERVES 4

**ONE POT/ONE PAN
FREEZER-FRIENDLY**

Prep time: 15 minutes

Cook time: 30 minutes

4 (5-ounce) skinless, boneless chicken breasts

½ teaspoon salt, divided

¼ teaspoon freshly ground black pepper, divided

1 cup unbleached all-purpose flour, plus 2 tablespoons

3 tablespoons olive oil, divided

10 ounces button mushrooms, thinly sliced

½ cup Marsala wine

½ cup low-sodium chicken broth

¼ cup cool water

1. Loosely wrap each chicken breast in plastic wrap and place on a cutting board. Using a mallet or heavy-bottomed pan, pound the chicken until each breast is about 1 inch thick. Unwrap the chicken and discard the plastic wrap.

2. Season both sides of the chicken with ¼ teaspoon of salt and ⅛ teaspoon of pepper.

3. Dredge both sides of the chicken in 1 cup of flour, shaking off any excess flour.

4. In a large skillet over medium heat, heat 2 tablespoons of olive oil. When the oil is shimmering, add the chicken breasts and cook for 10 minutes, flipping once, until browned on both sides. Remove from the pan and set aside.

5. Over medium heat, heat the remaining 1 tablespoon of olive oil. When the oil is shimmering, add the mushrooms and cook for 5 minutes, until softened. Add the wine and chicken broth, and bring the mixture to a boil. Reduce heat to medium-low and add the chicken breasts. Continue cooking, covered, for about 15 minutes, until the chicken reaches an internal temperature of 165°F.

6. In a small bowl, whisk together the remaining 2 tablespoons of flour and the water. Add the flour mixture to the skillet, and continue whisking until the mixture thickens, about 2 minutes.

CONTINUED

Chicken Marsala *continued*

7. Sprinkle the remaining ¼ teaspoon of salt and remaining
⅛ teaspoon of pepper, and toss to combine.

8. Serve warm or freeze for later. To freeze, place in a resealable
container in the freezer for up to 2 months. To defrost, refrigerate overnight. Reheat in a medium skillet over medium heat for
10 to 15 minutes. Reheat individual servings in the microwave on
high for 2 minutes.

TOBY'S TIP: Marsala is a sweet white wine and is usually sold at your local
market. You can substitute the Marsala with ½ cup dry white wine and
2 teaspoons brandy.

Serving size: 1 chicken breast plus ½ cup sauce
Per serving: Calories: 414; Total fat: 14g; Saturated fat: 2g; Protein: 37g;
Carbohydrates: 26g; Fiber: 1g; Sodium: 440mg

Chicken Enchilada Casserole

GLUTEN-FREE

I love Mexican fare but the calories can get out of control. Order enchiladas, and you can be talking close to 1,000 calories! That's without the bottomless tortilla chips and that must-have bowl of guac. This simple version is 550 per serving and *muy* satisfying.

SERVES 4

FREEZER-FRIENDLY

Prep time: 20 minutes

Cook time: 40 minutes

Cooking spray

8 ounces Easy Sautéed Chicken Breast (page 118) or rotisserie chicken, cut into bite-size pieces

1 (15-ounce) can low-sodium black beans

¼ teaspoon salt

⅛ teaspoon freshly ground black pepper

2½ cups Simple Salsa (page 189) or jarred salsa

12 corn tortillas

1½ cups shredded reduced-fat Cheddar cheese or Mexican cheese blend

1. Preheat the oven to 350°F. Coat an 8-by-12-inch baking dish with cooking spray.

2. In a medium bowl, combine the chicken and black beans. Add the salt and pepper, and toss to blend.

3. Spread ½ cup salsa on the bottom of the prepared baking dish. Top with 4 corn tortillas, slightly overlapping each other. Top with half of the chicken mixture, then ¾ cup salsa and ½ cup cheese. Top with another 4 corn tortillas and repeat with the chicken, salsa, and cheese. Top the casserole with the remaining 4 tortillas and cover evenly with the remaining ½ cup salsa and ½ cup cheese.

4. Bake for 40 minutes, until cheese is bubbling.

5. Cut the casserole into 4 pieces and serve warm, or freeze for later. To freeze, place cooled casserole in a freezer-safe container in the freezer for up to 2 months. To defrost, refrigerate overnight. Reheat, covered, in a 350°F oven for 20 to 25 minutes, until heated through.

TOBY'S TIP: Make your casserole vegetarian by swapping the chicken for sautéed onions, peppers, and brown rice.

Serving size: 1 piece
Per serving: Calories: 540; Total fat: 18g; Saturated fat: 6g; Protein: 36g; Carbohydrates: 61g; Fiber: 13g; Sodium: 849mg

Slow Cooker Rosemary-Lemon Chicken with Potatoes and Carrots

GLUTEN-FREE | DAIRY-FREE

Every time I went to my Grandma Rachel's house, she served up chicken and potatoes. I asked my father about this tradition, and he explained that when he was growing up, that was all she served to him as well. This dish is an ode to my Grandma Rachel.

SERVES 6

SLOW COOKER
FREEZER-FRIENDLY

Prep time: 15 minutes
Cook time: 4 hours on high or
7 hours on low

2 pounds baby red
potatoes, halved

1 cup baby carrots

1½ pounds skinless, boneless
chicken breasts

½ teaspoon salt, divided

¼ teaspoon freshly ground
black pepper, divided

1 cup low-sodium
chicken broth

1 tablespoon chopped
fresh rosemary

3 garlic cloves, minced

1. Spread the potatoes and carrots on the bottom of a slow cooker.

2. Season both sides of the chicken with ¼ teaspoon of salt and ⅛ teaspoon of pepper.

3. Place the chicken over the vegetables. Pour in the broth and add the rosemary, garlic, remaining ¼ teaspoon salt, and remaining ⅛ teaspoon pepper.

4. Cook on high for 4 hours or on low for 7 hours.

5. Serve immediately or freeze for later. To freeze, place cooled chicken, vegetables, and liquid in a resealable container or several containers in the freezer for up to 2 months. To defrost, refrigerate overnight. To reheat on the stovetop, bring the liquid to a boil and then lower the heat to medium and simmer until heated through. Alternatively, reheat in the oven at 375°F for 15 to 20 minutes. Individual portions can be reheated in the microwave on high for 2 to 3 minutes.

TOBY'S TIP: Add hard veggies that hold up well in a slow cooker, like parsnips, turnips, sweet potatoes, and yams.

Serving size: 4 ounces chicken plus ¾ cup vegetables
Per serving: Calories: 255; Total fat: 3g; Saturated fat: 1g; Protein: 29g; Carbohydrates: 27g; Fiber: 3g; Sodium: 389mg

Slow Cooker Pineapple Chicken

DAIRY-FREE

When I started dating, I would always suggest meeting at my favorite Malaysian restaurant for dinner. The service was quick, and if I wasn't interested in the company, at least I knew I was in for a good meal. The delicious pineapple chicken stuck with me through all these years, and now I whip it up in my slow cooker.

SERVES 8

SLOW COOKER
FREEZER-FRIENDLY

Prep time: 10 minutes

Cook time: 3 hours on high or 6 hours on low

1½ cups low-sodium chicken broth

¼ cup brown sugar

¼ cup low-sodium soy sauce

3 garlic cloves, minced

3 cups cubed fresh pineapple

2 pounds skinless, boneless chicken thighs

1. In a small bowl, whisk together the chicken broth, brown sugar, soy sauce, and garlic.

2. Add the pineapple to the bottom of a slow cooker. Top with the chicken, and drizzle with the broth mixture.

3. Cook on high for 3 hours or on low for 6 hours.

4. Serve the chicken and pineapple, discarding the excess liquid.

TOBY'S TIP: Swap out the pineapple for mango for a fun variation.

Serving size: 4 ounces chicken plus ¼ cup pineapple
Per serving: Calories: 418; Total fat: 25g; Saturated fat: 7g; Protein: 27g; Carbohydrates: 19g; Fiber: 1g; Sodium: 742mg

Turkey Bolognese

This easy dish is a staple in my house. When my kids get hungry, they can simply spoon it over whole-grain pasta and warm it in the microwave. Serve it with my Mediterranean Chopped Salad (page 41) for a complete meal.

SERVES 4

ONE POT/ONE PAN
FREEZER-FRIENDLY

Prep time: 10 minutes

Cook time: 30 minutes

1 tablespoon olive oil

1 onion, chopped

2 garlic cloves, minced

1 pound ground
turkey breast

1 (28-ounce) can
crushed tomatoes

½ cup dry white wine

2 teaspoons dried oregano

½ teaspoon salt

¼ teaspoon freshly
ground black pepper

1. In a medium saucepan over medium heat, heat the olive oil. When the oil is shimmering, add the onion and cook until translucent, about 3 minutes. Add the garlic and cook until fragrant, 1 minute more.

2. Add the ground turkey and cook for 5 minutes, breaking up the pieces with the back of a wooden spoon, until brown on all sides.

3. Add the crushed tomatoes and wine, and bring the mixture to a boil. Reduce heat and simmer, covered, for 20 minutes, until the flavors combine. Add the oregano, salt, and pepper, and stir to incorporate.

4. Serve warm or freeze for later. To freeze, place cooled sauce into a resealable container in the freezer for up to 2 months. To defrost, refrigerate overnight. Reheat the sauce in a medium saucepan over medium-high heat for 10 to 15 minutes, or reheat single-serve batches in the microwave on high for 2 minutes.

TOBY'S TIP: For even more flavor, add 2 or 3 bay leaves to the sauce before cooking, then remove them before serving.

Serving size: 1 cup
Per serving: Calories: 316; Total fat: 18g; Saturated fat: 4g; Protein: 23g; Carbohydrates: 18g; Fiber: 5g; Sodium: 727mg

Indian-Style Turkey Breast

GLUTEN-FREE

Garam masala is a blend of spices commonly used in Indian cuisine. It's typically made from a combo of black peppercorns, mace, nutmeg, cinnamon, cardamom, bay leaf, cumin, and coriander. Garam masala adds a warm, sweet flavor to poultry, lamb, fish, rice dishes, and potatoes.

SERVES 4

FREEZER-FRIENDLY

Prep time: 15 minutes, plus 30 minutes to marinate

Cook time: 10 minutes

1½ cups nonfat plain Greek yogurt, divided

2 teaspoons curry powder

1 teaspoon garam masala

1 teaspoon cayenne pepper

¼ teaspoon salt

⅛ teaspoon freshly ground black pepper

1¼ pounds skinless, boneless turkey breast cutlets

Cooking spray

1. In a large bowl, mix together 1 cup of yogurt with the curry powder, garam masala, cayenne, salt, and pepper.

2. Add the turkey cutlets to the yogurt marinade, and toss to evenly coat. Cover and refrigerate for 30 minutes to 1 hour.

3. Coat a grill pan with cooking spray and heat over medium heat. Shake off the excess marinade from the turkey cutlets and place them in the hot pan, leaving space between each cutlet. Discard the marinade. Cook the turkey for 4 minutes on each side, until cooked through.

4. Serve with the remaining ½ cup of Greek yogurt for dipping. To freeze, place cooled turkey in a resealable container in the freezer for up to 2 months. To defrost, refrigerate overnight. Reheat in a nonstick skillet or grill pan over medium heat for several minutes on each side, or reheat individual pieces in the microwave on high for about 1 minute.

TOBY'S TIP: Look for turkey breast cutlets in the poultry aisle or ask your local butcher. A full boneless turkey breast weighs around 2 pounds, but you can ask your butcher to cut the amount you need.

Serving size: 4 ounces turkey plus 2 tablespoons Greek yogurt
Per serving: Calories: 204; Total fat: 2g; Saturated fat: 0g; Protein: 41g; Carbohydrates: 4g; Fiber: 0g; Sodium: 675mg

Slow Cooker Turkey Breast with Onions

GLUTEN-FREE | DAIRY-FREE | PALEO-FRIENDLY

Who says you need to fuss over a whole turkey on Thanksgiving? If you're serving only a few people, why not let the slow cooker cook it up? This delicious, simple version incorporates a few spices, onion, garlic, and chicken broth, and is only 154 calories per serving.

SERVES 8

**SLOW COOKER
FREEZER-FRIENDLY**

Prep time: 10 minutes

Cook time: 4 hours on high or 8 hours on low

2 pounds skinless, boneless turkey breast

1 tablespoon olive oil

½ teaspoon salt

¼ teaspoon freshly ground black pepper

1 onion, sliced

3 garlic cloves, sliced

1 cup low-sodium chicken broth or turkey broth

1 teaspoon dried thyme

½ teaspoon paprika

1. Brush both sides of the turkey breast with the olive oil, and season with the salt and pepper.

2. Place the onion, garlic, and turkey breast in the slow cooker. Top with the broth, thyme, and paprika, and stir to combine.

3. Cook on high for 4 hours or on low for 8 hours.

4. Serve warm or freeze for later. To freeze, place cooled turkey breast with the liquid in a resealable container in the freezer for up to 2 months. To defrost, refrigerate overnight. Reheat in a 375°F oven for about 20 minutes, or reheat single-serve batches in the microwave on high for 2 minutes.

TOBY'S TIP: Pair this dish with Slow Cooker Cranberry Sauce (page 190).

Serving size: 4 ounces turkey plus ¼ of the onions
Per serving: Calories: 154; Total fat: 3g; Saturated fat: 1g; Protein: 27g; Carbohydrates: 2g; Fiber: 0g; Sodium: 351mg

Slow Cooker Turkey Chili

GLUTEN-FREE | DAIRY-FREE

Every Sunday night I make sure my kids and I sit down for a family dinner. Even still, Sundays tend to be very busy with parties, basketball games, and gymnastics tournaments, so this is when I love to use my slow cooker. Chili is the slow cooker family favorite, especially during the colder months.

SERVES 4

**SLOW COOKER
FREEZER-FRIENDLY**

Prep time: 15 minutes

Cook time: 4 hours

1 pound ground
turkey breast

2 (15-ounce) cans
low-sodium cannellini beans
or other white beans,
drained and rinsed

2 garlic cloves, minced

2 cups low-sodium
chicken broth

2 teaspoons ground cumin

1 teaspoon chili powder

¼ teaspoon salt

⅛ teaspoon freshly ground
black pepper

1. In a slow cooker, add the ground turkey, breaking up any chunks with the back of a spoon. Add the beans, garlic, broth, cumin, chili powder, salt, and pepper, and toss to incorporate. Cover and cook on low for 4 hours.

2. Serve warm or freeze. To freeze, place cooled chili in a resealable container in the freezer for up to 2 months. To defrost, refrigerate overnight. Reheat on the stovetop over medium-high heat for about 15 minutes, or reheat single-serve batches in the microwave on high for 3 minutes.

TOBY'S TIP: This chili is made with a chicken broth base, but you can swap the broth for 1 (28-ounce) can crushed tomatoes. If you want more veggies, use harder ones, like potatoes and carrots, which hold up well in the slow cooker.

Serving size: 1¼ cups

Per serving: Calories: 382; Total fat: 16g; Saturated fat: 4g; Protein: 30g; Carbohydrates: 30g; Fiber: 8g; Sodium: 582mg

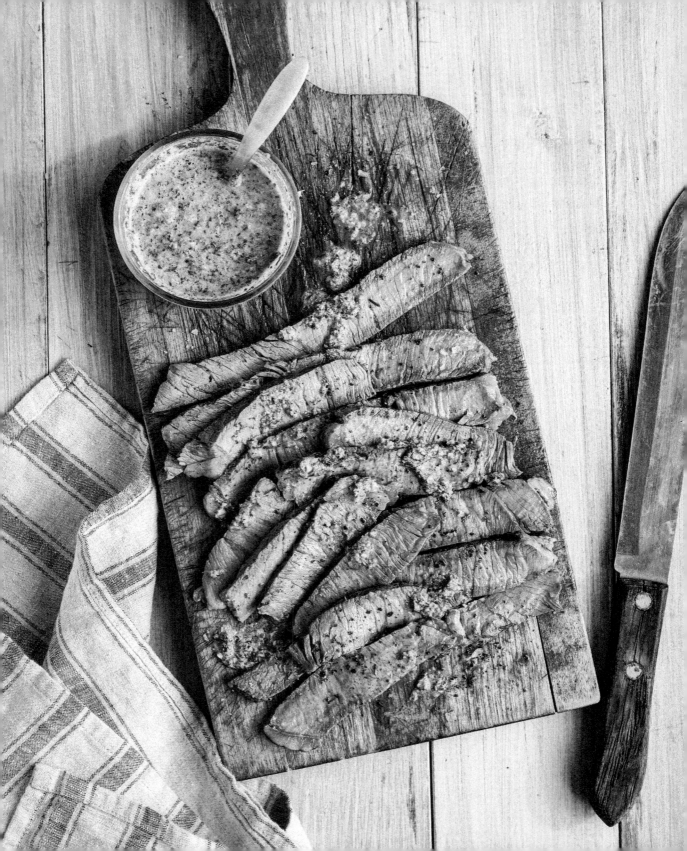

9

Beef and Pork Mains

Basic Meatballs

DAIRY-FREE

When I'm in a pinch, I whip up a comforting batch of meatballs with this very basic recipe. When it's served with a side of whole-grain pasta and my Mediterranean Chopped Salad (page 41), I know my family is getting the nutrition we need.

SERVES 4

30-MINUTE
FREEZER-FRIENDLY

Prep time: 15 minutes

Cook time: 15 minutes

1 pound 90% lean ground beef

1 onion, finely chopped

1 garlic clove, minced

1 large egg, beaten

¼ cup Homemade Bread Crumbs (page 192) or store-bought unseasoned bread crumbs

1 tablespoon Italian seasoning

½ teaspoon salt

¼ teaspoon freshly ground black pepper

2 tablespoons olive oil

1. In a large bowl, combine the ground beef, onion, garlic, egg, bread crumbs, Italian seasoning, salt, and pepper. Use clean hands to mix until well blended.

2. Shape 1 tablespoon of the meatball mixture into a ball, and place on a large plate. Repeat with the remaining mixture to make about 20 meatballs.

3. In a large skillet over medium heat, heat the olive oil. When the oil is shimmering, add the meatballs and cook, covered, about 15 minutes, browning on all sides until a thermometer inserted into a meatball reads 155°F.

4. Serve warm or freeze for later. To freeze, store cooled meatballs in a freezer-safe container in the freezer for up to 2 months. To defrost, refrigerate overnight. Reheat meatballs in a saucepan along with some Basic Tomato Sauce (page 184): Bring the sauce to a boil, then lower and simmer for 10 to 15 minutes until the meatballs are warmed through. Single-serve portions can be reheated in the microwave on high for about 2 minutes.

TOBY'S TIP: Italian seasoning is a combination of dried herbs, like oregano, basil, rosemary, thyme, and marjoram. You can easily swap out the Italian seasoning for ½ cup of any chopped fresh herb or a combination of them.

Serving size: About 5 meatballs

Per serving: Calories: 269; Total fat: 15g; Saturated fat: 5g; Protein: 26g; Carbohydrates: 6g; Fiber: 1g; Sodium: 427mg

Olive and Feta Burgers

I like getting creative with my burgers. Some days I feel like Mexican flavors, so I'll top them with avocado and salsa, while other days, I make these Mediterranean-style bad boys with olives and feta cheese, and top them with my Tahini Yogurt Sauce (page 186).

SERVES 4

30-MINUTE

Prep time: 15 minutes

Cook time: 15 minutes

1 pound 90% lean ground beef

½ cup crumbled feta cheese

½ cup pitted Kalamata olives, chopped

1 garlic clove, minced

1 large egg, beaten

¼ cup Homemade Bread Crumbs (page 192) or store-bought unseasoned bread crumbs

¼ teaspoon freshly ground black pepper

2 tablespoons olive oil

1. In a large bowl, combine the ground beef, feta, olives, garlic, egg, bread crumbs, and pepper.

2. Use clean hands to evenly divide the mixture into 4 burger patties.

3. In a large skillet or grill pan over medium-high heat, heat the olive oil. When the oil is shimmering, add the patties and cook for 3 to 5 minutes on each side, until browned and cooked through.

TOBY'S TIP: For burgers, meatloaf, and meatball recipes, stick with 90% lean ground beef. You need some fat to keep these babies moist!

Serving size: 1 burger

Per serving: Calories: 325; Total fat: 21g; Saturated fat: 8g; Protein: 28g; Carbohydrates: 5g; Fiber: 1g; Sodium: 388mg

Meatloaf in a Pinch

DAIRY-FREE

Every time someone serves me a slice of meatloaf, I find it dry, and I renew my vow to never serve anyone a dry slice. This meatloaf is brimming with moisture and flavor, thanks to a special ingredient—my Homemade Barbecue Sauce (page 187).

SERVES 8

FREEZER-FRIENDLY

Prep time: 15 minutes

Cook time: 1 hour

Cooking spray

1½ pounds 90% lean ground beef

1 cup Homemade Barbecue Sauce (page 187) or store-bought barbecue sauce, divided

¾ cup quick-cooking oats

1 onion, finely chopped

1 garlic clove, minced

1 large egg, beaten

½ teaspoon salt

¼ teaspoon freshly ground black pepper

1. Preheat the oven to 350°F. Coat a 9-by-5-inch loaf pan with cooking spray.

2. In a large bowl, add the ground beef, ½ cup of barbecue sauce, and the oats, onion, garlic, egg, salt, and pepper. Use clean hands to mix until well combined.

3. Place the meat mixture into the prepared loaf pan, making sure the top is level. Pour the remaining ½ cup of barbecue sauce over the meatloaf, using a spatula or the back of a wooden spoon to evenly spread it.

4. Bake for about 1 hour, until a thermometer inserted into the center of the meatloaf reads 155°F.

5. Remove from the oven, and allow to cool for 10 minutes. Cut into 8 equal slices.

6. Serve warm or freeze for later. To freeze, store cooled meatloaf sliced in a freezer-safe container in the freezer for up to 2 months. To defrost, refrigerate overnight. Reheat individual portions in the microwave on high for 1 to 1½ minutes.

TOBY'S TIP: To make this meatloaf gluten-free, use gluten-free oats and gluten-free barbecue sauce.

Serving size: 1 slice
Per serving: Calories: 244; Total fat: 10g; Saturated fat: 4g; Protein: 19g; Carbohydrates: 18g; Fiber: 1g; Sodium: 546mg

Skirt Steak Fajitas

GLUTEN-FREE | DAIRY-FREE | PALEO-FRIENDLY

One of my favorite dishes to order at a Mexican restaurant is steak fajitas. The entire experience is jump-started when the server brings my sizzling fajitas to the table. However, I have often found the amount served to be overwhelming, especially with the wide array of sides, which can jack up the calories to over 1,000! Luckily, I can easily whip up a healthy version at home, and serve it with the sides I choose in order to keep calories under 500 per serving.

SERVES 4

**ONE POT/ONE PAN
FREEZER-FRIENDLY**

Prep time: 15 minutes,
plus 30 minutes to marinate

Cook time: 15 minutes

2 tablespoons olive oil

1 garlic clove, minced

1½ teaspoons
smoked paprika

½ teaspoon ground cumin

½ teaspoon salt, divided

¼ teaspoon freshly ground
black pepper, divided

1¼ pounds skirt steak

Cooking spray

2 yellow bell peppers, seeded
and cut into ¼-inch strips

1 large onion, thinly sliced

1. In a large bowl, whisk the olive oil, garlic, paprika, cumin, ¼ teaspoon of salt, and ⅛ teaspoon of pepper. Add the skirt steak and toss to evenly coat. Cover the bowl and marinate in the refrigerator for at least 30 minutes and up to overnight.

2. Coat a large grill pan with cooking spray and heat over medium-high heat. Add the skirt steak and cook for 8 to 12 minutes, turning once, until it reaches an internal cooking temperature of 145°F.

3. Remove the steak from the grill pan and transfer to a cutting board to cool for 5 minutes.

4. Coat the grill pan again with cooking spray. Add the peppers and onion, and cook for about 5 minutes, until the vegetables soften.

5. Meanwhile, cut the steak into 1-inch strips.

6. Add the steak strips and the remaining ¼ teaspoon of salt and remaining ⅛ teaspoon of pepper to the pan with the vegetables, and toss to combine.

CONTINUED

7. Serve warm or freeze for later. To freeze, place cooled meat and vegetables in a resealable container in the freezer for up to 2 months. To defrost, refrigerate overnight. Reheat on the stove-top over medium heat for 8 to 10 minutes, until heated through. Individual portions can be reheated in the microwave on high for 1½ to 2 minutes.

TOBY'S TIP: Enjoy your fajitas in a whole-wheat tortilla, over a salad, or over my Black Beans and Farro (page 62).

Serving size: About 1¼ cups

Per serving: Calories: 367; Total fat: 25g; Saturated fat: 8g; Protein: 30g; Carbohydrates: 7g; Fiber: 2g; Sodium: 355mg

Grilled Steak with Herb Sauce

You don't have to go to a restaurant to have a good steak. Although beef has a reputation for being high in fat, about half the fatty acids in beef are monounsaturated, the same kind found in olive oil. So fire up your outdoor grill or indoor grill pan, and cook a delicious, mouthwatering steak whenever the mood strikes!

SERVES 4

30-MINUTE

Prep time: 10 minutes

Cook time: 20 minutes

Cooking spray

1 (1¼-pound) sirloin steak

½ teaspoon salt

⅛ teaspoon freshly ground black pepper

1 cup roughly chopped fresh cilantro leaves and stems

2 tablespoons capers, drained

2 scallions, roughly chopped

2 tablespoons olive oil

¼ cup water

Juice of 1 lemon

1 garlic clove, minced

1. Preheat the oven to 400°F. Coat an ovenproof grill pan or skillet with cooking spray.

2. Sprinkle both sides of the steak with the salt and pepper.

3. Heat the prepared grill pan over high heat. When the pan is hot, add the steak and cook on each side for 2 minutes. Place the pan in the oven and roast for about 12 minutes, until the steak reaches an internal temperature of 145°F.

4. Remove from the oven and transfer the steak to a cutting board to rest for 5 minutes.

5. Meanwhile, in a blender, add the cilantro, capers, scallions, olive oil, water, lemon juice, and garlic, and blend until almost smooth but still a little chunky.

6. Thinly slice the steak, and serve with the herb sauce.

TOBY'S TIP: Browning both sides of a steak in a skillet is called pan searing, which helps seal in the juices and forms a mouthwatering crust.

Serving size: 4 ounces steak plus 2 tablespoons sauce
Per serving: Calories: 335; Total fat: 23g; Saturated fat: 7g; Protein: 30g; Carbohydrates: 2g; Fiber: 0g; Sodium: 493mg

Beef Tenderloin with Red Wine Reduction

GLUTEN-FREE | PALEO-FRIENDLY

One of the most fun ways to spend time in the kitchen is making a red wine reduction. Pour a little wine in the pan, and while the sauce is simmering, go on and take a few swigs for yourself!

SERVES 4

Prep time: 10 minutes

Cook time: 30 minutes

Cooking spray

4 (5-ounce) beef tenderloin steaks

½ teaspoon salt, divided

¼ teaspoon freshly ground black pepper, divided

1 cup dry red wine

1 shallot, finely chopped

1 tablespoon tomato paste

½ cup low-sodium beef broth

1. Coat a grill pan with cooking spray and heat over medium heat.

2. Sprinkle the steaks with ¼ teaspoon of salt and ⅛ teaspoon of pepper.

3. When the cooking spray is shimmering, place the steaks in the pan and cook for 7 to 10 minutes, turning once, until a thermometer inserted into the thickest part reads 145°F. Transfer the steaks to a platter.

4. In a small saucepan, add the wine, shallot, and tomato paste, and bring to a boil. Reduce heat and simmer for 8 minutes, stirring occasionally, until the liquid is reduced by about half. Add the beef broth and return the mixture to a boil. Reduce heat and simmer for another 8 minutes, until the liquid is again reduced by about half. Add the remaining ¼ teaspoon of salt and remaining ⅛ teaspoon of pepper, and stir to combine.

5. Top each steak with 3 tablespoons of the red wine reduction.

TOBY'S TIP: Want a smoother reduction? Strain it and throw away the solids. You can enjoy your red wine reduction either way.

Serving size: 1 steak plus 3 tablespoons sauce
Per serving: Calories: 230; Total fat: 10g; Saturated fat: 4g; Protein: 31g; Carbohydrates: 3g; Fiber: 1g; Sodium: 425mg

Slow Cooker Shredded Barbecue Beef

DAIRY-FREE

Fuel your body with an array of easy lean beef recipes throughout the week. With increased trimming practices, there are more than 30 cuts of beef that qualify as lean. Lean beef has dynamite nutrition, loaded with 10 essential nutrients and fewer calories than you think.

SERVES 6

SLOW COOKER
FREEZER-FRIENDLY

Prep time: 15 minutes

Cook time: 6 to 8 hours

1 (4-pound) pot roast, like bottom round

½ cup Homemade Barbecue Sauce (page 187) or bottled barbecue sauce

½ cup low-sodium beef broth

1. Place the pot roast in a slow cooker and cover with the barbecue sauce and beef broth. Using the back of a wooden spoon or spatula, spread the barbecue sauce over the pot roast. Cover and cook on low for 6 to 8 hours, until a thermometer inserted into the center of the roast reads 145°F.

2. Remove the roast and transfer to a plate, reserving the sauce. Allow the roast to cool for 10 minutes.

3. Using two forks, shred the beef and place into a large bowl. Add the reserved sauce and toss to coat.

4. Serve warm or freeze for later. To freeze, store cooled beef in a freezer-safe container in the freezer for up to 2 months. To defrost, refrigerate overnight. Reheat in a saucepan over medium heat for 5 to 10 minutes, until the beef and sauce are warmed through. Single-serve portions can be reheated in the microwave on high for about 1½ minutes.

TOBY'S TIP: Serve this dish over polenta, Black Beans and Farro (page 62), or a baked potato. You can also make quesadillas using the shredded beef and some cheese.

Serving size: 1 cup

Per serving: Calories: 434; Total fat: 13g; Saturated fat: 5g; Protein: 67g; Carbohydrates: 8g; Fiber: 0g; Sodium: 464mg

Slow Cooker Beef with Bell Peppers

Bell peppers are packed with phytochemicals, which are plant compounds linked to good health and disease prevention. Zeaxanthin and chlorogenic acid are two phytochemicals linked to cancer prevention, while lycopene is a powerful antioxidant that helps lower the risk of heart disease, prostate cancer, and macular degeneration.

SERVES 6

SLOW COOKER
FREEZER-FRIENDLY

Prep time: 10 minutes

Cook time: 6 to 8 hours

1 (2-pound) top round steak or London broil

½ teaspoon salt

¼ teaspoon freshly ground black pepper

1 large onion, thinly sliced

2 red bell peppers, seeded and cut into ¼-inch strips

¾ cup Basic Tomato Sauce (page 184) or jarred tomato sauce

½ cup low-sodium beef broth

1. Season the steak with the salt and pepper, and place in the slow cooker. Top with the onion, peppers, tomato sauce, and broth. Stir to combine.

2. Cover and cook on low for 6 to 8 hours, until the beef reaches an internal cooking temperature of 145°F.

3. Cut the steak into thin slices and serve warm or freeze for later. To freeze, place cooled steak with vegetables and liquid into a resealable container in the freezer for up to 2 months. To defrost, refrigerate overnight. Reheat in a large skillet on the stovetop for about 10 minutes, or reheat individual portions in the microwave on high for about 2 minutes.

TOBY'S TIP: Serve this dish over quinoa or brown rice, or roll it into a whole-wheat tortilla.

Serving size: 4 ounces steak plus about ½ cup vegetables

Per serving: Calories: 248; Total fat: 9g; Saturated fat: 3g; Protein: 34g; Carbohydrates: 6g; Fiber: 2g; Sodium: 386mg

Pork Larb

This Asian dish is made from ground meat and flavored with lime juice, cilantro, mint, red pepper flakes, and anchovy paste. The tart, spicy, and salty flavor balances beautifully with the fresh herbs.

SERVES 4

30-MINUTE

Prep time: 10 minutes

Cook time: 15 minutes

1 tablespoon olive oil

1 pound ground pork

¼ cup Thai Dressing (page 183)

3 shallots, thinly sliced

½ cup chopped fresh cilantro

24 Bibb lettuce leaves

1. In a medium skillet over medium heat, heat the olive oil. When the oil is shimmering, add the ground pork and cook for 10 to 12 minutes, until browned, using a wooden spoon to break it up. Remove from heat and drain any liquid. Allow the pork to cool for 10 minutes.

2. Pour the Thai Dressing into a medium bowl. Add the cooked pork and toss to blend. Add the shallots and cilantro, and gently stir to incorporate.

3. Scoop 2 tablespoons of the meat into each of 24 lettuce leaves. Serve warm.

TOBY'S TIP: You can swap the ground pork for ground turkey.

Serving size: 6 pieces
Per serving: Calories: 402; Total fat: 33g; Saturated fat: 8g; Protein: 22g; Carbohydrates: 6g; Fiber: 1g; Sodium: 131mg

Herbed Pork Meatballs

DAIRY-FREE

There are two ways I like to whip up a batch of meatballs. The first is on the stovetop, where I use only 2 tablespoons of olive oil to cook them up. I also like to bake the meatballs in a mini-muffin tin at 350°F for about 25 minutes. To keep them moist, I store them in my Basic Tomato Sauce (page 184).

SERVES 4

30-MINUTE
FREEZER-FRIENDLY

Prep time: 15 minutes
Cook time: 15 minutes

1 pound ground pork

1 onion, finely chopped

1 garlic clove, minced

1 large egg, beaten

½ cup whole-wheat panko bread crumbs

½ cup finely chopped fresh parsley

½ teaspoon salt

¼ teaspoon freshly ground black pepper

2 tablespoons olive oil

1. In a large bowl, combine the ground pork, onion, garlic, egg, bread crumbs, parsley, salt, and pepper.

2. Shape 1 tablespoon of the pork mixture into a ball, and place on a large plate. Repeat with the remaining mixture to make about 20 meatballs.

3. In a large skillet over medium heat, heat the olive oil. When the oil is shimmering, add the meatballs and cook, covered, for about 15 minutes, browning on all sides until a thermometer inserted into a meatball reads 155°F.

4. Serve warm or freeze for later. To freeze, store cooled meatballs in a resealable container in the freezer for up to 2 months. To defrost, refrigerate overnight. Reheat the meatballs in a saucepan along with Basic Tomato Sauce (page 184): Bring the sauce to a boil, then lower and simmer for 10 to 15 minutes until the meatballs are warmed through. Single-serve portions of meatballs can be reheated in the microwave on high for about 2 minutes.

TOBY'S TIP: Add more herbs to the mix, using any combination of parsley, sage, rosemary, or thyme.

Serving size: About 5 meatballs
Per serving: Calories: 365; Total fat: 26g; Saturated fat: 7g; Protein: 23g; Carbohydrates: 9g; Fiber: 1g; Sodium: 406mg

Asian-Spiced Pork Loin

DAIRY-FREE

Chinese five-spice powder is a delicious combination of cinnamon, cloves, fennel seed, star anise, and peppercorns. These warming flavors merge with the spiciness of cayenne and the sweetness of brown sugar, which together create a mouthwatering complement to this pork loin.

SERVES 8

FREEZER-FRIENDLY

Prep time: 10 minutes, plus 30 minutes to marinate

Cook time: 50 minutes

⅓ cup low-sodium soy sauce

2 garlic cloves, minced

3 tablespoons Chinese five-spice powder

2 tablespoons light brown sugar

1 teaspoon cayenne pepper

½ teaspoon salt

1 (2-pound) pork loin, fat trimmed

Cooking spray

1. In a medium bowl, whisk together the soy sauce, garlic, Chinese five-spice powder, brown sugar, cayenne, and salt. Add the pork loin, and turn to evenly coat. Cover the bowl and marinate in the refrigerator for at least 30 minutes or up to overnight.

2. Preheat the oven to 400°F. Coat a baking sheet with cooking spray.

3. Transfer the pork to the baking sheet, discarding the marinade. Bake for 40 to 50 minutes, until a thermometer inserted into the thickest part of the loin reads 145°F.

4. Remove from the oven, and transfer to a cutting board to cool for 10 minutes. Cut into ¾-inch-thick slices.

5. Serve warm or freeze for later. To freeze, store cooled pork in a freezer-safe container in the freezer for up to 2 months. To defrost, refrigerate overnight. Reheat several slices in the microwave on high for 1 to 2 minutes.

TOBY'S TIP: Pick up Chinese five-spice powder in the Asian section of your supermarket, or if you're feeling creative, make your own!

Serving size: 4 ounces pork
Per serving: Calories: 164; Total fat: 5g; Saturated fat: 2g; Protein: 25g; Carbohydrates: 5g; Fiber: 0g; Sodium: 502mg

Pork Tenderloin with Apple-Tarragon Sauce

GLUTEN-FREE | DAIRY-FREE

If you're looking to grow your own herbs, tarragon is an easy one to start with. It will last all summer and through the fall. Tarragon has feathery leaves and has an element of anise flavor, which complements fruits (like these apples) beautifully in protein dishes.

SERVES 4

ONE POT/ONE PAN
30 MINUTES

Prep time: 5 minutes
Cook time: 25 minutes

1 tablespoon olive oil

1 (1¼-pound) pork tenderloin

2 medium apples, cored and sliced

1 tablespoon unsalted butter

2 garlic cloves, minced

2 cups apple cider vinegar

½ teaspoon salt

⅛ teaspoon freshly ground black pepper

2 teaspoons chopped fresh tarragon

1. Preheat the oven to 400°F.

2. In a large ovenproof skillet over medium heat, heat the olive oil. When the oil is shimmering, add the pork tenderloin and cook about 8 minutes, turning occasionally, until browned on all sides.

3. Add the apple slices, and place the skillet in the oven. Bake for about 20 minutes, until the pork reaches a minimum internal temperature of 145°F. Place the pork on a cutting board to cool for 5 minutes. Transfer the apples to a plate, and set aside.

4. Carefully return the skillet to the stovetop over medium heat, and add the butter. When the butter is melted, add the garlic and cook until fragrant, 1 minute. Add the apple cider vinegar, and use a wooden spoon to scrape the pork bits from the bottom of the pan. Bring the mixture to a boil, then reduce heat and simmer for 2 minutes, until the flavors combine. Add the salt, pepper, and tarragon, and stir to incorporate. Turn off the heat.

5. Thinly slice the cooled pork tenderloin, then return it to the skillet. Add the apples and toss to evenly coat. Transfer to a serving dish and serve warm.

TOBY'S TIP: Do you like your sauce thicker? Whisk ¼ cup water with 2 tablespoons cornstarch, then add it to the sauce when it is simmering. After a few minutes, you'll notice the sauce thicken.

Serving size: About 5 ounces pork plus 1¼ cups sauce
Per serving: Calories: 256; Total fat: 9g; Saturated fat: 3g; Protein: 29g; Carbohydrates: 13g; Fiber: 2g; Sodium: 641mg

Miso-Garlic Pork Chops

GLUTEN-FREE | DAIRY-FREE

Miso is made from fermented soybeans. This thick paste adds that special umami flavor to dishes. When you think miso, soup may automatically pop into mind, but miso is also terrific in marinades and salad dressings.

SERVES 4

ONE POT/ONE PAN

Prep time: 10 minutes, plus 30 minutes to marinate

Cook time: 10 minutes

⅓ cup white miso

⅓ cup sake

⅓ cup mirin

2 teaspoons minced fresh ginger

1 garlic clove, minced

4 (5-ounce) boneless pork loin chops

Cooking spray, or 1 tablespoon olive oil

1. In a large bowl, mix the miso, sake, mirin, ginger, and garlic into a smooth paste.

2. Add the pork chops and turn to coat all sides with the glaze. Marinate in the refrigerator for at least 30 minutes or up to overnight.

3. Coat a grill pan with cooking spray and heat over medium heat. Alternatively, brush the grates of an outdoor grill with the olive oil. When the pan or grill is hot, cook the pork chops for about 3 to 5 minutes on each side, until they reach an internal cooking temperature of 145°F.

TOBY'S TIP: You can also use bone-in pork chops. The cook time depends not on whether it has a bone but on the thickness of the chop, which can vary from ½ inch to 2 inches. Either way, follow the cook time directed in the recipe, and use a thermometer to gauge doneness.

Serving size: 1 pork chop
Per serving: Calories: 209; Total fat: 4g; Saturated fat: 1g; Protein: 32g; Carbohydrates: 12g; Fiber: 1g; Sodium: 932mg

Slow Cooker Honey Mustard Pork with Pears

DAIRY-FREE

I like pairing proteins with fruit, as you can see from my Pork Tenderloin with Apple-Tarragon Sauce (page 150) and Slow Cooker Pineapple Chicken (page 131). It helps increase my daily fruit and phytochemical intake, and the taste profile drives my taste buds crazy.

SERVES 8

**SLOW COOKER
FREEZER-FRIENDLY**

Prep time: 10 minutes

Cook time: 3 to 4 hours on high for 6 to 8 hours on low

¼ cup Homemade Honey Mustard (page 181)

⅓ cup low-sodium chicken broth

½ teaspoon salt

¼ teaspoon freshly ground black pepper

1 (2-pound) boneless pork loin, fat trimmed

2 pears, peeled, cored, and thinly sliced

1 tablespoon cornstarch

2 tablespoons water

1. In a small bowl, whisk together the honey mustard, broth, salt, and pepper.

2. Place the pork and pears in the slow cooker. Pour the honey mustard mixture over the top.

3. Cover and cook on high for 3 to 4 hours or on low for 6 to 8 hours.

4. Remove the pork from the slow cooker, retaining the pears and liquid, and transfer to a cutting board to cool for 10 minutes, then thinly slice.

5. In a small bowl, whisk together the cornstarch and water.

6. In a medium skillet over medium heat, heat the pears and liquid from the slow cooker. Add the cornstarch mixture and continue whisking for about 3 minutes, until the mixture thickens.

7. Serve the pork slices topped with the warm sauce, or freeze for later. To freeze, store cooled pork in a freezer-safe container in the freezer for up to 2 months. To defrost, refrigerate overnight. Reheat in a saucepan over medium heat for 5 to 10 minutes, until the pork and sauce are warmed through. Single-serve portions can be reheated in the microwave on high for about 1½ minutes.

TOBY'S TIP: Add veggies to this dish by adding 1 to 2 cups of baby carrots to the slow cooker.

Serving size: About 4 ounces pork plus ½ cup pears with sauce
Per serving: Calories: 212; Total fat: 8g; Saturated fat: 2g; Protein: 24g; Carbohydrates: 9g; Fiber: 1g; Sodium: 368mg

Slow Cooker Cranberry Pork Chops

DAIRY-FREE

Although cranberries have a short season in the fall, cranberry farmers are busy throughout the year tending to their marshes. For example, in the winter, when there are long stretches of very cold days, farmers flood the cranberry beds with water to form ice that will coat the vines and keep them protected while they are dormant. Cranberry farmers don't have a lot of free time during off-harvest seasons, as they're always busy ensuring that the crop is taken care of; it's a 24/7/365 job.

SERVES 4

**SLOW COOKER
FREEZER-FRIENDLY**

Prep time: 10 minutes

Cook time: 3 hours on high or
6 hours on low

4 (5-ounce) boneless
pork chops

½ teaspoon salt

¼ teaspoon freshly ground
black pepper

1 onion, thinly sliced

1½ cups fresh or thawed
frozen cranberries

½ cup apple juice

¼ cup balsamic vinegar

2 tablespoons honey

1. Season both sides of the pork chops with the salt and pepper.

2. In a slow cooker, add the pork chops, onion, and cranberries.

3. In a small bowl, whisk together the apple juice, balsamic vinegar, and honey. Pour over the pork chops.

4. Cover and cook on high for 3 hours or on low for 6 hours.

5. Serve warm or freeze for later. To freeze, store cooled pork chops with the sauce in a freezer-safe container in the freezer for up to 2 months. To defrost, refrigerate overnight. Reheat the pork chops and sauce in a saucepan over medium-high heat for about 10 minutes. Alternatively, reheat individual pork chops with sauce in the microwave on high for about 2 minutes.

TOBY'S TIP: Fresh cranberries are in season from October through December. You can find frozen cranberries all year round in the freezer aisle.

Serving size: 1 pork chop plus ½ cup sauce
Per serving: Calories: 278; Total fat: 10g; Saturated fat: 3g; Protein: 24g; Carbohydrates: 21g; Fiber 2g; Sodium: 361mg

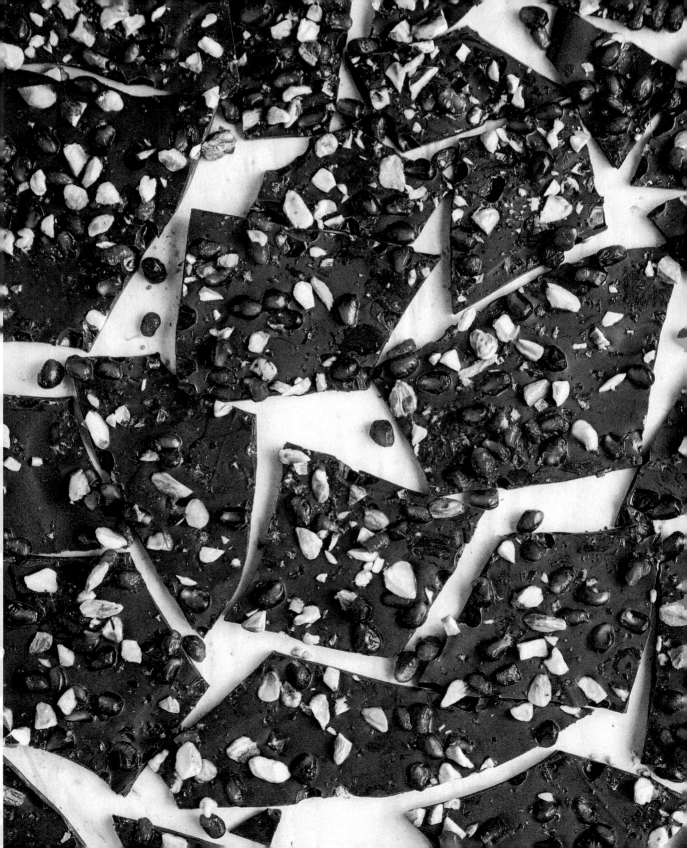

10 Desserts and Sweet Treats

Homemade Caramel-Dipped Apples

GLUTEN-FREE | VEGETARIAN

When I was growing up, my Grandpa Jack owned a candy shop in Brooklyn, New York. Every time I went to visit him at work, the smell of burnt caramel from the caramel-dipped apples drew me in. Through the display glass, I would see the rows of caramel-dipped apples, some plain and others covered with peanuts, calling my name. To this day, anywhere I spot caramel apples, it immediately takes me back to these unforgettable childhood memories.

SERVES 4

30-MINUTE

Prep time: 10 minutes,
plus 15 minutes to chill

Cook time: 1 minute

Equipment: 4 wooden skewers

4 Pink Lady, Honeycrisp, Fuji, or Granny Smith apples

Cooking spray

½ cup Homemade Caramel Sauce (page 193)

½ cup unsalted peanuts, chopped

1. Remove the stems of the apples, and push a wooden skewer into the bottom of each apple, about three quarters of the way through.

2. Line a baking sheet with parchment paper and coat with cooking spray.

3. Warm the caramel sauce in a microwave-safe bowl for 1 minute, stirring frequently.

4. Quickly roll each apple in the caramel sauce. Use a spoon to cover the apple with the sauce.

5. Roll or dip the caramel apples in the chopped nuts, then place on the prepared baking sheet. Refrigerate until the caramel hardens, about 15 minutes.

TOBY'S TIP: Choose firm apples, like the ones listed, that will stand up to the heat of the caramel sauce. Otherwise, they can lose their crunch.

Serving size: 1 caramel apple
Per serving: Calories: 311; Total fat: 16g; Saturated fat: 6g; Protein: 5g; Carbohydrates: 40g; Fiber: 6g; Sodium: 64mg

Coconut-Date Pudding

GLUTEN-FREE | DAIRY-FREE | PALEO-FRIENDLY

Store shelves are lined with the usual two pudding flavors: vanilla and chocolate. Sometimes you can find rice pudding. I find it frustrating not being able to find other, more interesting flavors to enjoy. That's why I make my own using a combo of milk, a little sweetener, and fun flavors. Dates give this pudding a naturally sweet flavor and combined with the crunchy walnuts, it's perfection in every bite.

SERVES 4

Prep time: 10 minutes, plus 3 hours to chill

Cook time: 10 minutes

Equipment: 4 (8-ounce) ramekins

3 cups unsweetened coconut milk, divided

1½ cups pitted Medjool dates, chopped

4 tablespoons (¼ cup) chopped walnuts

3 tablespoons water

1 teaspoon gelatin

1 teaspoon ground cinnamon

1. In a medium saucepan, bring 1 cup of coconut milk and the dates to a boil. Reduce heat to medium-low, and continue cooking, stirring often, until the liquid evaporates, about 5 minutes.

2. Divide the dates between the 4 ramekins, pressing them into the bottom. Top the dates in each ramekin with 1 tablespoon of walnuts.

3. Add the remaining 2 cups of coconut milk to the saucepan, and heat over medium heat.

4. In a small bowl, whisk the water and gelatin, then add to the saucepan. Bring to a boil, reduce heat to medium, and whisk for about 5 minutes, until the gelatin is incorporated. Add the cinnamon, stirring to blend. Remove from heat and allow to slightly cool.

5. Pour the coconut mixture evenly between the 4 ramekins. Loosely cover with plastic wrap, and refrigerate the puddings to set for at least 3 hours or up to overnight.

TOBY'S TIP: Once the puddings are set, punch up the flavor by sprinkling orange zest over the top of each.

Serving size: 1 pudding
Per serving: Calories: 334; Total fat: 10g; Saturated fat: 9g; Protein: 5g; Carbohydrates: 67g; Fiber: 8g; Sodium: 46mg

Strawberry Compote in Red Wine Syrup

GLUTEN-FREE | DAIRY-FREE | VEGAN | VEGETARIAN

Dress up fresh fruit with a drizzle of delicious, warming syrup. The sweet wine, spiked with a hint of vanilla and cinnamon, is the perfect ending to any meal.

SERVES 4

30-MINUTE

Prep time: 10 minutes

Cook time: 20 minutes

1 cup red wine

⅓ cup granulated sugar

1 teaspoon vanilla extract

½ teaspoon ground cinnamon

4 cups strawberries, hulled and sliced

1. In a medium saucepan, bring the wine, sugar, vanilla, and cinnamon to a boil. Reduce heat and simmer until the liquid is reduced by half, about 20 minutes.

2. Place 1 cup of berries into each of 4 cups. Drizzle with 2 tablespoons of the red wine syrup.

3. Serve warm or chill in the refrigerator before serving.

TOBY'S TIP: Substitute the strawberries for whatever's in season—sliced peaches, plums, pitted cherries, raspberries, or blackberries.

Serving size: 1 cup

Per serving: Calories: 119; Total fat: 0g; Saturated fat: 0g; Protein: 1g; Carbohydrates: 28g; Fiber: 3g; Sodium: 2mg

Milk Chocolate Peanut Butter Cups

Although everyone is always talking about how much they love dark chocolate, my taste buds don't agree. I'm a "super taster," which means that to me, dark chocolate tastes extra bitter. I prefer the milk variety, but I do swap it out for dark chocolate in many recipes or use a combo of dark and milk chocolate. Whichever you choose, chocolate can be enjoyed in small amounts in a healthy diet.

SERVES 12

Prep time: 10 minutes, plus 1 hour to chill

Cook time: 5 minutes

Cooking spray

12 ounces milk chocolate, broken into pieces

2 tablespoons coconut oil

12 teaspoons natural creamy peanut butter

⅛ teaspoon sea salt

1. Spray 12 mini-muffin liners with cooking spray, then place in an 8-by-8 dish.

2. In a small saucepan, bring a cup of water to a boil, then reduce heat to a simmer. Fit a heat-proof medium bowl on top of the saucepan to make a double boiler. Add the chocolate and coconut oil to the bowl, stirring gently with a wooden spoon until smooth, about 5 minutes.

3. Fill one-third of each muffin liner with melted chocolate, then 1 teaspoon of peanut butter, and top with melted chocolate.

4. Transfer the dish to the refrigerator and allow to set for at least 1 hour.

TOBY'S TIP: Use 60% dark chocolate or a combination of dark and milk chocolate.

Serving size: 1 peanut butter cup
Per serving: Calories: 194; Total fat: 12g; Saturated fat: 7g; Protein: 3g; Carbohydrates: 21g; Fiber: 1g; Sodium: 66mg

Pomegranate-Pistachio Bark

GLUTEN-FREE | DAIRY-FREE | PALEO-FRIENDLY | VEGAN | VEGETARIAN

One year I threw a holiday party, and a guest brought some killer white chocolate bark. I couldn't get enough, and neither could most of the guests, as it was the talk of the party. Ever since then, I've been experimenting with all types of chocolate and toppings, and here's one of my favorites.

MAKES 24 PIECES

Prep time: 10 minutes, plus 45 minutes to chill

Cook time: 10 minutes

½ cup raw shelled pistachios, roughly chopped

1 pound 60% dark chocolate, broken into pieces

½ cup pomegranate arils, liquid drained

⅛ teaspoon sea salt

1. Line a baking sheet with parchment paper. Set aside.

2. Heat a small skillet over medium heat. Add the pistachios and cook until toasted, about 3 minutes. Set aside to cool.

3. In a small saucepan, bring a cup of water to a boil, then reduce heat to a simmer. Place a heat-proof medium bowl on top of the saucepan to make a double boiler. Add the chocolate to the bowl and cook, stirring gently with a wooden spoon until the mixture is smooth, about 5 minutes. Spoon the chocolate onto the prepared baking sheet, spreading to the edges evenly with a spatula.

4. Evenly sprinkle the chocolate with the pistachios, pomegranate arils, and sea salt.

5. Transfer the baking sheet to the refrigerator for about 45 minutes, until the chocolate sets.

6. Break the bark into 24 pieces and serve.

TOBY'S TIP: Sprinkle your own fun combination over the melted chocolate. You can try walnuts and dried cherries, toasted coconut flakes and almonds, or dried bananas and toasted pecans.

Serving size: 1 piece

Per serving: Calories: 127; Total fat: 8g; Saturated fat: 4g; Protein: 2g; Carbohydrates: 11g; Fiber: 2g; Sodium: 13mg

Chocolate-Dipped Citrus Fruit

GLUTEN-FREE | DAIRY-FREE | PALEO-FRIENDLY | VEGAN | VEGETARIAN

When it's in season, I stock up on citrus fruit and place the bowl front and center on my kitchen counter. That way, every time my kids or I pass the bowl, we have a juicy, vitamin C–rich fruit staring us in the face. This recipe takes citrus in a different direction for a special treat.

SERVES 10

Prep time: 15 minutes, plus 15 minutes to chill

Cook time: 5 minutes

4 ounces 60% dark chocolate, broken into pieces

1 tablespoon coconut oil

3 clementines, peeled and segmented

1 navel orange, peeled and segmented

3 mandarin oranges, peeled and segmented

1. Line a baking sheet with parchment paper.

2. In a small saucepan, bring about a cup of water to a boil, then reduce heat to a simmer. Place a heat-proof medium bowl on top of the saucepan to make a double boiler. Add the chocolate and coconut oil, and stir gently with a wooden spoon until the mixture is smooth, about 5 minutes.

3. One at a time, dip the tip of each citrus segment into the melted chocolate, and place onto the prepared baking sheet, leaving about ½ inch between pieces.

4. Place in the refrigerator to set, about 15 minutes.

TOBY'S TIP: Experiment with citrus! Different varieties of citrus are available throughout the year, including Cara Cara oranges, blood oranges, pummelos, red grapefruits, Minneola tangelos, and golden nugget mandarins.

Serving size: 5 pieces

Per serving: Calories: 92; Total fat: 5g; Saturated fat: 3g; Protein 1g; Carbohydrates: 11g; Fiber: 2g; Sodium: 1mg

Banana-Cinnamon "Ice Cream"

GLUTEN-FREE | DAIRY-FREE | VEGAN | VEGETARIAN

It's amazing how frozen bananas can transform into a perfect, creamy, dairy-free dessert. Savor the cold, sweet flavor after your meal, or enjoy as a snack any time of day.

SERVES 4

ONE POT/ONE PAN
30-MINUTE
FREEZER-FRIENDLY

Prep time: 10 minutes

4 medium frozen bananas, cut into 2-inch chunks

¼ cup 100% maple syrup

1 teaspoon ground cinnamon

1. Allow the frozen banana chunks to rest at room temperature for 5 minutes, then place in a food processor or blender.

2. Add the maple syrup and cinnamon, and purée until well combined.

3. Serve immediately, or store in a freezer-safe container in the freezer until later.

TOBY'S TIP: Purée the frozen bananas with 2 tablespoons of Homemade Caramel Sauce (page 193) for banana-caramel "ice cream"!

Serving size: ½ cup
Per serving: Calories: 159; Total fat: 0g; Saturated fat: 0g; Protein: 1g; Carbohydrates: 41g; Fiber: 3g; Sodium: 4mg

Berry Yogurt Trifle

VEGETARIAN

The gorgeous red, white, and blue colors that are displayed in this trifle scream "summer," which makes this treat especially perfect for your Fourth of July, Memorial Day, or Labor Day celebration.

SERVES 8

Prep time: 15 minutes, plus 30 minutes to chill

2 cups nonfat vanilla Greek yogurt

2 tablespoons honey

1 (10-ounce) store-bought angel food cake, cut into 1-inch cubes

1½ cups strawberries, hulled and halved

1½ cups blueberries

1 cup Vanilla-Infused Whipped Cream (page 194)

1. In a small bowl, mix together the yogurt and honey.

2. In a large bowl or trifle dish, distribute half of the angel food cake in an even layer. Top the cake with 1 cup of the yogurt mixture, using a spatula to evenly coat. Top with half of the strawberries and blueberries. Repeat to make a second layer, then top with the whipped cream.

3. Cover and refrigerate to set, about 30 minutes.

TOBY'S TIP: For an exclusively grown-up spin, spike your trifle by mixing the berries in a little Grand Marnier.

Serving size: ⅛ trifle

Per serving: Calories: 243; Total fat 6g; Saturated fat: 4g; Protein: 8g; Carbohydrates: 41g; Fiber: 2g; Sodium: 291mg

Honey-Peach Ice Pops

Many ice pop brands found in the frozen aisle are packed with added sugar, additives, and colors. Instead, you can whip up your own 60-calorie brand in 10 minutes, and they're filled with ingredients you can feel good about.

SERVES 6

FREEZER-FRIENDLY

Prep time: 10 minutes,
plus 4 hours to freeze

Equipment: 6 ice pop molds

1¼ cups diced fresh or
thawed frozen peaches

1 cup nonfat vanilla
Greek yogurt

2 tablespoons
100% maple syrup

¼ cup 2% fat milk

2 teaspoons freshly
squeezed lemon juice

½ teaspoon ground
cinnamon

1. In a blender, add the peaches, yogurt, syrup, milk, lemon juice, and cinnamon, and blend until smooth.

2. Using a ¼-cup scoop, pour the purée into the ice pop molds, and top each with a stick.

3. Freeze until set, at least 4 hours.

TOBY'S TIP: For a delicious surprise in each ice pop, place a peach slice inside each empty mold before filling it with the liquid mixture.

Serving size: 1 ice pop
Per serving: Calories: 63; Total fat: 0g; Saturated fat: 0g; Protein: 3g; Carbohydrates: 12g; Fiber: 1g; Sodium: 18mg

Ellena's Peanut Butter Cookies

GLUTEN-FREE | DAIRY-FREE | VEGETARIAN

These cookies combine my daughter Ellena's two favorite things: peanut butter and baking. She'll eat peanut butter any time of day: on bread, with fruit, or in yogurt. My girl is also obsessed with baking, and she makes cupcakes, cookies, and cakes whenever she can. I created these cookies on her behalf.

MAKES 14 COOKIES

Prep time: 15 minutes

Cook time: 20 minutes

Cooking spray

1 cup packed light brown sugar

1 large egg

1 teaspoon vanilla extract

1 cup natural creamy peanut butter

⅛ teaspoon salt

1. Preheat the oven to 350°F. Coat a baking sheet with cooking spray.

2. In a medium bowl, whisk together the brown sugar, egg, and vanilla.

3. Add the peanut butter and salt, mixing well to combine.

4. Scoop out 1 teaspoon of the batter, and use clean hands to roll into a ball. Place on the prepared baking sheet, pressing down to flatten. Repeat with the remaining batter, leaving ½ inch between cookies.

5. Bake on the center rack in the oven for 18 to 20 minutes, until the cookies are golden brown.

6. Remove from the oven and allow the cookies to cool for 5 minutes. Transfer the cookies to a wire rack to finish cooling for at least 10 minutes before serving.

TOBY'S TIP: Add chopped peanuts to the batter for even more peanut flavor.

Serving size: 1 cookie

Per serving: Calories: 173; Total fat: 9g; Saturated fat: 2g; Protein: 4g; Carbohydrates: 20g; Fiber: 1g; Sodium: 118mg

Flourless Double-Chocolate Chip Cookies

GLUTEN-FREE | DAIRY-FREE | VEGETARIAN

The healthy unsaturated fat in these cookies comes from the almond butter, which also gives these gluten-free babies their body. With its combination of chocolate chips and cocoa powder, one of these double-chocolate treats is all you'll need to curb a sweet tooth.

MAKES 15 COOKIES

30-MINUTE

Prep time: 15 minutes

Cook time: 15 minutes

Cooking spray

1 cup creamy almond butter

6 tablespoons honey

1 tablespoon unsweetened cocoa powder

2 large eggs

½ teaspoon salt

⅓ cup semisweet chocolate chips

1. Preheat the oven to 350°F. Coat a baking sheet with cooking spray.

2. In a blender, add the almond butter, honey, cocoa powder, eggs, and salt, and blend until smooth. Fold in the chocolate chips.

3. Scoop out 1 teaspoon of batter, and use clean hands to form into a ball. Place on the prepared baking sheet, pressing to flatten into a disc. Repeat with the remaining batter, leaving 1 inch between cookies.

4. Bake on the center rack in the oven for 12 to 15 minutes, until the cookies are golden brown.

5. Remove from the oven and allow the cookies to cool for 5 minutes. Transfer to a wire rack to finish cooling for at least 10 minutes before serving.

TOBY'S TIP: Swap the chocolate chips for dried tart cherries or dried cranberries.

Serving size: 1 cookie
Per serving: Calories: 159; Total fat: 11g; Saturated fat: 1g; Protein: 5g; Carbohydrates: 13g; Fiber: 2g; Sodium: 88mg

Almond Macaroons

GLUTEN-FREE | VEGETARIAN

Every Passover, my mother serves macaroons because they contain no wheat, unlike flour-based recipes. Now that I'm in my own home, macaroons have become a staple dessert I like to serve on holidays.

MAKES 16 MACAROONS

30-MINUTE

Prep time: 15 minutes

Cook time: 15 minutes

1 (7-ounce) package unsweetened coconut flakes

⅔ cup sweetened condensed milk

⅓ cup raw almonds, finely chopped

¼ cup honey

1 teaspoon almond extract

3 egg whites

1. Preheat the oven to 350°F. Line a baking sheet with parchment paper.

2. In a medium bowl, add the coconut, milk, almonds, honey, and almond extract, and stir to combine.

3. In another medium bowl, add the egg whites. Using an electric hand mixer, beat the egg whites until soft peaks form.

4. Gently fold the beaten egg whites into the coconut mixture.

5. Spoon out 1 heaping tablespoon of the mixture. Use clean hands to roll into a ball and place on the prepared baking sheet. Continue with the remainder of the batter, leaving about 1 inch between macaroons.

6. Bake for 12 to 15 minutes, until the macaroons are slightly browned.

TOBY'S TIP: For a chocaholic take on macaroons, melt some dark chocolate in the microwave. Drizzle the chocolate over cooled macaroons or dip each macaroon in the chocolate.

Serving size: 1 macaroon
Per serving: Calories: 164; Total fat: 11g; Saturated fat: 8g; Protein: 3g; Carbohydrates: 16g; Fiber: 2g; Sodium: 30mg

Banana-Oat Walnut Loaf

GLUTEN-FREE | DAIRY-FREE | VEGETARIAN

My daughters love the banana bread mix sold at Trader Joe's. Although I'm a big fan of the supermarket chain, I like to make my bread from scratch. This combo of whole grains, fruit, and nuts means that my kids are getting three different food groups; plus, my girls and I have more fun making it together when there's a little more to do.

SERVES 8

FREEZER-FRIENDLY

Prep time: 15 minutes

Cook time: 25 minutes

Cooking spray

2 cups gluten-free rolled oats, plus 2 tablespoons

3 ripe bananas, mashed

2 large eggs, lightly beaten

½ cup honey

1 teaspoon baking soda

½ cup raw walnuts, chopped

1. Preheat the oven to 350°F. Coat an 8-inch loaf pan with cooking spray.

2. In a medium bowl, mix together 2 cups of oats and the mashed bananas, beaten eggs, honey, and baking soda. Gently fold in the walnuts.

3. Pour the mixture into the prepared pan, spreading in an even layer with a spatula. Sprinkle the remaining 2 tablespoons of oats on top of the batter.

4. Bake for about 25 minutes, until the top is golden brown and a toothpick inserted into the center comes out clean. Remove from the oven and allow to cool for 10 minutes. Transfer the bread to a wire rack and let cool for 10 to 15 more minutes, then cut into 1-inch slices.

5. To freeze, place each slice in a resealable plastic bag or wrap them individually in plastic wrap and store the slices in the freezer for up to 2 months. To defrost, refrigerate overnight. The loaf can be eaten at room temperature, warmed in a toaster oven, or reheated in the microwave on high for 20 to 30 seconds. Allow the slices to cool for 2 minutes after reheating in the microwave before eating.

TOBY'S TIP: For a balanced breakfast, serve this Banana-Oat Walnut Loaf with nonfat plain Greek yogurt or a glass of skim or low-fat milk.

Serving size: 1 slice

Per serving: Calories: 205; Total fat: 6g; Saturated fat: 1g; Protein: 4g; Carbohydrates: 36g; Fiber: 3g; Sodium: 122mg

Quick Chocolate Cake

VEGETARIAN

Sometimes you just want a good old chocolate cake made from butter, flour, sugar, and eggs. Oftentimes, however, these desserts come with a supersized caloric price tag, racking up close to 1,000 calories per serving. This dessert comes in at 300 calories, so you can still indulge while skipping the guilt.

SERVES 8

Prep time: 15 minutes

Cook time: 25 minutes

Cooking spray

4 ounces semisweet chocolate, broken into pieces

6 tablespoons (¾ stick) unsalted butter, cut into pieces

¾ cup granulated sugar

3 large eggs

1 cup unbleached all-purpose flour

1. Preheat the oven to 425°F. Coat an 8-inch round cake pan with cooking spray.

2. In a microwave-safe bowl, add the chocolate and butter on high at 30-second intervals, stirring between each interval, until smooth, about 2 minutes.

3. Using an electric mixer, mix the sugar and eggs until the mixture thickens. Add the flour and continue to mix until combined. Add the chocolate mixture, and mix to incorporate.

4. Pour the batter into the prepared cake pan, and bake for 22 to 25 minutes, until a toothpick inserted into the cake comes out clean.

5. Remove from the oven and allow to cool for at least 15 minutes. Cut into 8 pieces and serve.

TOBY'S TIP: Go nuts by adding 1/2 cup chopped walnuts to the batter.

Serving size: 1 piece
Per serving: Calories: 303; Total fat: 15g; Saturated fat: 9g; Protein: 5g; Carbohydrates: 39g; Fiber: 1g; Sodium: 28mg

Applelicious Apple Crisp

VEGETARIAN

I opt for apple crisp over apple pie, as it has a fraction of the calories. A modest slice of apple pie weighs in at over 400 calories and 20 grams of fat—and that's without the ice cream! My crisp has all the applelicious flavor but one-third fewer calories and 65 percent less fat.

SERVES 6

Prep time: 15 minutes

Cook time: 40 minutes

FOR THE FILLING

Cooking spray

6 medium apples (like Empire, Honeycrisp, Pink Lady), cored and thinly sliced

2 tablespoons honey

FOR THE TOPPING

¾ cup old-fashioned oats

¾ cup whole-wheat pastry flour

⅓ cup light brown sugar

3 tablespoons unsalted butter, at room temperature, cut into pieces

3 tablespoons water

1. Preheat the oven to 350°F. Coat an 8-by-8-inch baking dish with cooking spray.

2. Place the apples in a medium bowl. Add the honey and toss to coat. Transfer to the prepared baking dish.

3. To make the topping, in a blender, add the oats, flour, brown sugar, butter, and water, and blend until smooth.

4. Use clean fingers to crumble the topping over the apples.

5. Place the baking dish in the middle rack of the oven, and bake for 40 minutes, until the topping is browned and the apples are cooked through.

6. Remove from the oven and allow to cool for at least 10 minutes. Using a spoon, divide the crisp into six portions and serve.

TOBY'S TIP: Bruised apples give off an ethylene gas that promotes ripening, which may cause foods around them to spoil. Store apples at room temperature, or for a longer shelf life, store in the refrigerator in a brown paper bag. Use bruised or aging apples immediately.

Serving size: ⅙th of crisp

Per serving: Calories: 268; Total fat: 7g; Saturated fat: 4g; Protein: 3g; Carbohydrates: 51g; Fiber: 6g; Sodium: 2mg

Slow Cooker Poached Pears with Pomegranate Sauce

GLUTEN-FREE | DAIRY-FREE | VEGAN | VEGETARIAN

Impress guests with this simple yet elegant dessert. They'll think you languished in the kitchen, but only you'll know the work was all done simply by pressing the "On" button.

SERVES 4

SLOW COOKER

Prep time: 15 minutes

Cook time: 1½ hours

4 pears, peeled, halved, and cored

1½ cups 100% pomegranate juice

3 tablespoons flavored vodka (optional)

2 tablespoons 100% maple syrup

½ teaspoon ground cinnamon

1. Place the pears, cut-side down, in the slow cooker.

2. In a small bowl, whisk together the pomegranate juice, vodka (if using), syrup, and cinnamon, and pour over the pears.

3. Cover and cook on low until the pear is fork-soft, about 90 minutes.

TOBY'S TIP: Ripen pears at room temperature, and press with your thumb at the stem to check for ripeness. If it gives to gentle pressure, it is ripe and ready to eat. You can refrigerate ripe pears to keep them for several more days.

Serving size: 2 pear halves plus 3 tablespoons sauce
Per serving: Calories: 181; Total fat: 1g; Saturated fat: 0g; Protein: 1g; Carbohydrates: 46g; Fiber: 6g; Sodium: 11mg

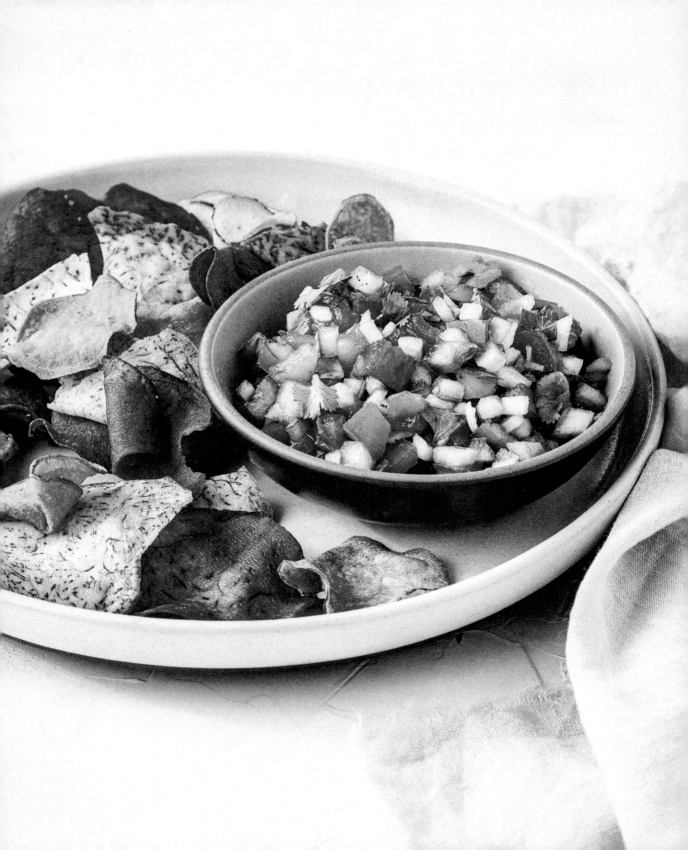

Sauces, Dressings, and Staples

Balsamic Vinaigrette

GLUTEN-FREE | DAIRY-FREE | VEGAN | VEGETARIAN

Although it's one of the most basic dressings, this is one of my favorites. It's the first dressing I learned how to make when I attended the food and nutrition program at New York University. My food science class met weekly in a test kitchen, and this particular class taught the concept of emulsifying oil and vinegar. It's a simple, tasty dressing well worth sharing.

MAKES 1 CUP

**ONE POT/ONE PAN
30-MINUTE**

Prep time: 10 minutes

¼ cup balsamic vinegar

1 teaspoon gluten-free Dijon mustard

½ teaspoon salt

¼ teaspoon freshly ground black pepper

¾ cup olive oil

1. In a small bowl, whisk together the vinegar, mustard, salt, and pepper. Slowly drizzle the olive oil into the mixture, and whisk to incorporate.

2. Store in the refrigerator for up to 2 weeks.

TOBY'S TIP: This dressing pairs well with many salads, including Kale and Green Cabbage Salad (page 42), White Bean and Arugula Salad (page 46), and Green Salad with Poached Salmon (page 47).

Serving size: 2 tablespoons
Per serving: Calories: 187; Total fat: 20g; Saturated fat: 3g; Protein: 0g; Carbohydrates: 2g; Fiber: 0g; Sodium: 165mg

Raspberry Vinaigrette

GLUTEN-FREE | DAIRY-FREE | VEGAN | VEGETARIAN

When I was single, I lived in a 350-square-foot apartment on New York's Upper East Side. I didn't have much of a kitchen, but always felt decadent whenever I had a bottle of mouth-puckering raspberry vinaigrette in the refrigerator. Now that I make my own, I can have a batch in my refrigerator any time I like.

MAKES ½ CUP

ONE POT/ONE PAN
30-MINUTE

Prep time: 10 minutes

⅓ cup frozen
raspberries, thawed

1 tablespoon red
wine vinegar

Juice of 1 lemon

1 teaspoon granulated sugar

¼ teaspoon salt

⅛ teaspoon freshly ground
black pepper

6 tablespoons olive oil

1. In a blender, add the raspberries, red wine vinegar, lemon juice, sugar, salt, and pepper, and blend until smooth. With the machine running, gradually add the olive oil and blend until incorporated.

2. Store in the refrigerator for up to 2 weeks.

TOBY'S TIP: Use this sweet-and-sour dressing to balance salads containing bitter greens, like arugula, spinach, and kale.

Serving size: 2 tablespoons
Per serving: Calories: 190; Total fat: 20g; Saturated fat: 2g; Protein: 0g; Carbohydrates: 2g; Fiber: 0g; Sodium: 150mg

Orange Dressing

In my family, my father is the fan of everything orange: chocolate-covered orange peel, orange dressing, orange marmalade—you name it! I never understood his obsession until I started tossing my salads with orange dressing. Now this orange dressing is an integral part of my healthy dressing repertoire.

MAKES ½ CUP

**ONE POT/ONE PAN
30-MINUTE**

Prep time: 10 minutes

Zest and juice of 1 orange

1 tablespoon
balsamic vinegar

1 teaspoon honey

¼ teaspoon salt

⅛ teaspoon freshly ground
black pepper

⅓ cup olive oil

1. In a blender, add the orange zest and juice, balsamic vinegar, honey, salt, and pepper, and blend until smooth. With the machine running, gradually add the olive oil and blend until incorporated.

2. Store in the refrigerator for up to 2 weeks.

TOBY'S TIP: You can also use this orange dressing as a marinade for chicken or fish.

Serving size: 2 tablespoons
Per serving: Calories: 174; Total fat: 18g; Saturated fat: 2g; Protein: 0g; Carbohydrates: 4g; Fiber: 0g; Sodium: 149mg

Dijon Dressing

GLUTEN-FREE | DAIRY-FREE | PALEO-FRIENDLY | VEGETARIAN

Use this savory Dijon dressing to punch up the flavor of a salad or as a marinade for steak, lamb, or fish. One teaspoon of Dijon mustard has about 10 calories and a small amount of nutrients, including thiamine, magnesium, phosphorus, and selenium. It's a delicious way to boost the flavor of any dish for very few calories.

MAKES 1 CUP

ONE POT/ONE PAN
30-MINUTE

Prep time: 5 minutes

5 tablespoons red wine vinegar

4 teaspoons gluten-free Dijon mustard

4 teaspoons honey

1 garlic clove, minced

¼ teaspoon salt

⅔ cup extra-virgin olive oil

1. In a small bowl, whisk together the vinegar, mustard, honey, garlic, and salt.

2. While continuously whisking, slowly drizzle in the olive oil to incorporate.

3. Store in the refrigerator for up to 2 weeks.

TOBY'S TIP: To cut back on calories but not flavor, use 1 tablespoon per serving. That will come to 88 calories and 9.5 grams of fat per serving instead.

Serving size: 2 tablespoons
Per serving: Calories: 175; Total fat: 19g; Saturated fat: 3g; Protein: 0g; Carbohydrates: 4g; Fiber: 0g; Sodium: 137mg

Lighter Caesar Dressing

GLUTEN-FREE | DAIRY-FREE | PALEO-FRIENDLY

When I first got into eating healthy, I would order Caesar salad whenever I went out to eat. Little did I know that the dressing was often a calorie bomb! Now that I am in the know about what's *really* healthy, I was able to build my own flavorful Caesar dressing for a fraction of the calories.

MAKES ½ CUP

ONE POT/ONE PAN
30-MINUTE

Prep time: 5 minutes

1 garlic clove, minced

Zest and juice of 1 lemon

1 teaspoon yellow mustard

½ teaspoon anchovy paste

3 tablespoons olive oil

1. In a small bowl, whisk together the garlic, lemon zest and juice, mustard, and anchovy paste. Whisking continuously, slowly drizzle in the olive oil until well combined.

2. Store in the refrigerator for up to 2 weeks.

TOBY'S TIP: In most of the dressings in this chapter, you can swap the olive oil for extra-virgin olive oil or canola oil.

Serving size: 2 tablespoons
Per serving: Calories: 95; Total fat: 10g; Saturated fat: 1g; Protein: 0g; Carbohydrates: 1g; Fiber: 0g; Sodium: 63mg

Lighter Green Goddess Dressing

GLUTEN-FREE | VEGETARIAN

This lightened, gorgeously-hued dressing is made from a combination of flavorful, low-calorie herbs and creamy Greek yogurt. As a result, it only has 25 calories per serving.

SERVES 12

**ONE POT/ONE PAN
30-MINUTE**

Prep time: 10 minutes

Cook time: 0 minutes

½ cup nonfat plain
Greek yogurt

1 tablespoon nonfat milk

½ cup roughly chopped
fresh parsley

½ cup roughly chopped
fresh basil

1 shallot, roughly chopped

1 clove garlic, sliced

1 tablespoon freshly
squeezed lemon juice

½ teaspoon salt

⅛ teaspoon freshly ground
black pepper

1. In a blender, add the Greek yogurt, milk, parsley, basil, shallot, garlic, lemon juice, salt, and black pepper, and blend until smooth.

2. Store in the refrigerator for up to 1 week.

TOBY'S TIP: To help reduce food waste, use leftover fresh herbs like tarragon and chives in your Greek Goddess dressing.

Serving size: 2 tablespoons
Per serving: Calories: 25; Total fat: 0g; Saturated Fat: 0g; Protein 3g; Carbohydrates:3g; Fiber 1g; Sodium: 211mg

Better-for-You Blue Cheese Dressing

GLUTEN-FREE | VEGETARIAN

When I was in high school, my family owned a cheese store in New York City called Cheeses of All Nations. During the few years they owned the store, I had the opportunity to taste a whole lot of the 400 varieties. Today I am a hard-core cheese lover, but I don't love the calories that go along with it. Luckily, I've found a few cheese hacks, including the trick of adding a small amount of a potent cheese, like blue, into a dressing so you can get all the flavor without all the calories.

MAKES ½ CUP

**ONE POT/ONE PAN
30-MINUTE**

Prep time: 5 minutes

1 (5.3-ounce) container nonfat plain Greek yogurt

2 tablespoons (about 1 ounce) crumbled blue cheese

1 garlic clove, smashed

2 teaspoons white wine vinegar

2 teaspoons freshly squeezed lemon juice

¼ teaspoon salt

⅛ teaspoon freshly ground black pepper

1. In a blender or food processor, add the yogurt, cheese, garlic, vinegar, lemon juice, salt, and pepper. Blend until smooth and creamy.

2. Store in the refrigerator for up to 1 week.

TOBY'S TIP: This creamy, tart dressing pairs beautifully with spicy foods, like my Buffalo Chicken Skewers (page 64) and Sweet and Spicy Chicken Fingers (page 121)

Serving size: 2 tablespoons
Per serving: Calories: 47; Total fat: 2g; Saturated fat: 1g; Protein: 5g; Carbohydrates: 2g; Fiber: 0g; Sodium: 245mg

Homemade Honey Mustard

GLUTEN-FREE | DAIRY-FREE | VEGETARIAN

When I was a teenager, I discovered honey mustard. The combo of the spicy Dijon balanced with the sweet honey just made me swoon. It was my trademark condiment for many years, until I realized how many hidden ingredients some restaurants added to it, including bacon and corn syrup. Now I make a homemade version so I control the input, and I usually have all the ingredients hanging out in my pantry, which means no extra cost!

MAKES ¾ CUP

ONE POT/ONE PAN
30-MINUTE

Prep time: 5 minutes

⅓ cup reduced-fat mayonnaise

¼ cup gluten-free Dijon mustard

¼ cup honey

1 tablespoon white wine vinegar

¼ teaspoon cayenne pepper

¼ teaspoon salt

1. In a small bowl, whisk together the mayonnaise, mustard, honey, vinegar, cayenne, and salt.

2. Store in the refrigerator for up to 1 week.

TOBY'S TIP: There are many new types of mayonnaise you can choose from, including avocado based, canola based, olive oil based, and vegan. They may not come in a reduced-fat version but are all good options to use in this recipe.

Serving size: 2 tablespoons
Per serving: Calories: 103; Total fat: 5g; Saturated fat: 0g; Protein: 0g; Carbohydrates: 13g; Fiber: 0g; Sodium: 452mg

Goat Cheese Dressing

GLUTEN-FREE | VEGETARIAN

I adore creamy dressings, but not the hundreds of calories that accompany them. My trick for lightening up creamy dressings is to combine a small amount of a flavorful cheese with Greek yogurt, which carries the cheesy flavor beautifully for a fraction of the calories.

MAKES 1 CUP

ONE POT/ONE PAN
30-MINUTE

Prep time: 5 minutes

3 ounces crumbled goat cheese

¼ cup nonfat plain Greek yogurt

½ cup low-fat milk

Zest and juice of 1 lemon

1 scallion, chopped

¼ teaspoon salt

⅛ teaspoon freshly ground black pepper

1. In a blender, add the cheese, yogurt, milk, lemon zest and juice, scallion, salt, and pepper, and blend until smooth.

2. Store in the refrigerator for up to 1 week.

TOBY'S TIP: Swap the Greek yogurt for the same amount of reduced-fat sour cream.

Serving size: 2 tablespoons
Per serving: Calories: 52; Total fat: 3g; Saturated fat: 2g; Protein: 4g; Carbohydrates: 2g; Fiber: 0g; Sodium: 130mg

Thai Dressing

GLUTEN-FREE | DAIRY-FREE | PALEO-FRIENDLY

I like to keep a collection of different dressings and marinades on hand so I can use whichever I'm in the mood for. I'll make a double batch at the beginning of the week and then use it to make several dishes. This is a good one to enhance a variety of dishes (see Toby's Tip).

MAKES ½ CUP

**ONE POT/ONE PAN
30-MINUTE**

Prep time: 10 minutes

½ cup chopped fresh mint leaves

8 teaspoons toasted sesame oil

¼ cup olive oil

Zest and juice of 4 limes

⅛ teaspoon red pepper flakes

1 teaspoon anchovy paste

1. In a small bowl, whisk together the mint, sesame oil, olive oil, lime zest and juice, red pepper flakes, and anchovy paste.

2. Store in the refrigerator for up to 2 weeks.

TOBY'S TIP: This Thai Dressing can be used over salads or to marinate chicken, fish, pork, beef, or tofu.

Serving size: 1 tablespoon
Per serving: Calories: 104; Total fat: 12g; Saturated fat: 2g; Protein: 0g; Carbohydrates: 1g; Fiber: 0g; Sodium: 48mg

Basic Tomato Sauce

GLUTEN-FREE | DAIRY-FREE | PALEO-FRIENDLY | VEGAN | VEGETARIAN

Instead of purchasing jarred tomato sauce, you can make a healthier, tastier version in no time using canned tomatoes. Enjoy this tomato sauce with Snack Pizza with Chicken and Mushrooms (page 81), Spanish-Style Chicken in Tomato Sauce (page 123), and Turkey Bolognese (page 132).

MAKES 7 CUPS

ONE POT/ONE PAN
FREEZER-FRIENDLY

Prep time: 15 minutes

Cook time: 20 minutes

2 tablespoons olive oil

2 onions, chopped

4 garlic cloves, minced

2 (28-ounce) cans crushed tomatoes with basil

1 (6-ounce) can tomato paste

1 teaspoon dried oregano

½ teaspoon dried thyme

½ teaspoon salt

¼ teaspoon freshly ground black pepper

1. In a medium pot over medium heat, heat the olive oil. When the oil is shimmering, add the onions and cook for 3 minutes, until translucent. Add the garlic and cook until fragrant, 1 minute more.

2. Add the crushed tomatoes, tomato paste, oregano, thyme, salt, and pepper, and stir to combine. Bring to a boil, then reduce heat to medium-low. Cover and simmer for about 15 minutes, until the flavors combine.

3. To store, cool the tomato sauce, then refrigerate in a resealable container for up to 2 weeks or freeze. Freeze cooled tomato sauce in a freezer-safe container for up to 3 months. To defrost, refrigerate overnight. Reheat individual portions in the microwave on high for about 1 minute. A larger batch can be reheated in a saucepan over medium heat for 10 to 15 minutes.

TOBY'S TIP: BPA (bisphenol-A) is a synthetic compound found in many plastics and the lining of cans and thought to have negative health consequences. However, the Food and Drug Administration recently conducted a safety assessment of BPA and stated that the levels currently occurring in food are perfectly safe. Many companies, however, have removed it from their products. You can look for *BPA-free* on the label, but know that even though they may not all be labeled, 90 percent of canned tomatoes no longer contain BPA.

Serving size: ½ cup

Per serving: Calories: 39; Total fat: 1g; Saturated fat: 0g; Protein: 1g; Carbohydrates: 6g; Fiber: 1g; Sodium: 225mg

Easy Pesto Sauce

GLUTEN-FREE | DAIRY-FREE | PALEO-FRIENDLY | VEGAN | VEGETARIAN

The versatility of pesto sauce transcends pasta. Explore the options on pizza, fish, chicken, pork, or beef; drizzle it over eggs; whisk it into a salad dressing; or use it to garnish a soup. Although you may be worried about the fat, it's the healthy, unsaturated kind, which can be guiltlessly enjoyed in moderation.

MAKES ¾ CUP

ONE POT/ONE PAN
30-MINUTE

Prep time: 5 minutes

2 cups fresh basil

¼ cup olive oil

½ teaspoon salt

2 tablespoons freshly squeezed lemon juice

4 or 5 tablespoons water, as needed

1. In a blender, add the basil, olive oil, salt, and lemon juice. Add 4 tablespoons of cool water and purée. Add more water if needed to reach the desired consistency.

2. Store in the refrigerator for up to 1 week.

TOBY'S TIP: For an easy twist on traditional pesto, swap out the basil for spinach, arugula, or parsley.

Serving size: About 2 tablespoons
Per serving: Calories: 83; Total fat: 9g; Saturated fat: 1g; Protein: 0g; Carbohydrates: 1g; Fiber: 0g; Sodium: 198mg

Tahini Yogurt Sauce

GLUTEN-FREE | VEGETARIAN

As a young girl, I spent many summers in Israel. Tahini, or sesame seed paste, was part of our everyday dishes. It's added as an ingredient to hummus, made into a dressing to go with schnitzel (fried chicken breast), drizzled over falafel, or tucked inside lamb gyros. Tahini has become one of my go-to ingredients, especially in this unbelievably easy-to-make sauce.

MAKES 1 CUP

ONE POT/ONE PAN
30-MINUTE

Prep time: 5 minutes

1 cup nonfat plain Greek yogurt

¼ cup tahini

2 tablespoons freshly squeezed lemon juice

½ teaspoon salt

1. In a medium bowl, mix together the yogurt, tahini, lemon juice, and salt.

2. Store in the refrigerator for up to 1 week.

TOBY'S TIP: This Tahini Yogurt Sauce can accompany my Baked Lentil Falafel (page 86) or be used as a dip for crudité.

Serving size: 2 tablespoons
Per serving: Calories: 62; Total fat: 4g; Saturated fat: 1g; Protein: 4g; Carbohydrates: 3g; Fiber: 1g; Sodium: 160mg

Homemade Barbecue Sauce

DAIRY-FREE

Barbecue sauce is known to have hidden sugar. Although you need to add *some* sugar to get the delicious flavor, many bottled barbecue sauces add more than you really need. Making my own savory blend allows me to control the ingredients, especially that pesky added sugar.

MAKES ¾ CUP

ONE POT/ONE PAN
30-MINUTE

Prep time: 10 minutes

¾ cup ketchup

4 teaspoons apple cider vinegar

2 tablespoons brown sugar

1 tablespoon Worcestershire sauce

1 garlic clove, minced

2 teaspoons smoked paprika

⅛ teaspoon salt

1. In a small bowl, whisk together the ketchup, vinegar, brown sugar, Worcestershire sauce, garlic, paprika, and salt.

2. Store in the refrigerator for up to 2 weeks.

TOBY'S TIP: Use this sauce for Slow Cooker Shredded Barbecue Beef (page 145) and Meatloaf in a Pinch (page 140).

Serving size: 2 tablespoons
Per serving: Calories: 51; Total fat: 0g; Saturated fat: 0g; Protein: 1g; Carbohydrates: 12g; Fiber: 0g; Sodium: 333mg

Soy-Ginger Sauce

DAIRY-FREE | VEGAN | VEGETARIAN

Say goodbye to the dubious bottled stuff, and hello to simple sauces using five ingredients. I love to control the ingredients while saving money. Look in your pantry—all those bottled marinades and sauces cost several dollars each!

MAKES ½ CUP

ONE POT/ONE PAN
30-MINUTE

Prep time: 5 minutes

4 teaspoons low-sodium soy sauce

1 tablespoon toasted sesame oil

1 tablespoon grated fresh ginger

1 tablespoon cornstarch

¼ cup cool water

⅛ teaspoon red pepper flakes

1. In a small bowl, whisk together the soy sauce, sesame oil, ginger, cornstarch, water, and red pepper flakes.

2. Store in the refrigerator for up to 2 weeks.

TOBY'S TIP: Substitute ¼ teaspoon ground ginger for 1 tablespoon of grated fresh ginger.

Serving size: 2 tablespoons
Per serving: Calories: 42; Total fat: 4g; Saturated fat: 1g; Protein: 0g; Carbohydrates: 3g; Fiber: 0g; Sodium: 107mg

Simple Salsa

GLUTEN-FREE | DAIRY-FREE | PALEO-FRIENDLY | VEGAN | VEGETARIAN

My kids are addicted to chips and salsa. Instead of buying endless jars of salsa, I started making my own. I can make it as spicy as I want by adding a jalapeño pepper, or I can keep it as is (which is the mild version).

MAKES 2½ CUPS

**ONE POT/ONE PAN
30-MINUTE**

Prep time: 15 minutes

5 plum tomatoes, chopped (about 1 pound)

½ green bell pepper, seeded and chopped

½ small onion, chopped

¼ cup chopped fresh cilantro

Juice of 1 lime

1 tablespoon olive oil

½ teaspoon salt

¼ teaspoon freshly ground black pepper

1. In a medium bowl, add the tomatoes, bell pepper, onion, and cilantro. Mix to combine. Add the lime juice, olive oil, salt, and pepper, and mix to evenly coat.

2. Store in the refrigerator for up to 1 week.

TOBY'S TIP: To make a smooth salsa, place the ingredients in a blender or use an immersion blender and blend until smooth.

Serving size: ¼ cup
Per serving: Calories: 23; Total fat: 1g; Saturated fat: 0g; Protein: 1g; Carbohydrates: 3g; Fiber: 1g; Sodium: 62mg

Slow Cooker Cranberry Sauce

During the hustle and bustle of Thanksgiving, I am most thankful for any recipe that uses a slow cooker—here's one of them. I just take a few minutes to toss the ingredients into that bad boy and press *Cook* so I can get back to preparing the rest of the dishes in the kitchen. When my timer goes off, I know I'll have a delicious cranberry sauce that everyone at the table will be gushing over.

MAKES 4 CUPS

SLOW COOKER

Prep time: 15 minutes

Cook time: 4 hours

Juice of 2 oranges and zest of 1 orange

Juice of 2 lemons and zest of 1 lemon

½ cup water

⅛ teaspoon ground cloves

½ cup 100% maple syrup

2 (12-ounce) packages (6 cups) fresh or frozen cranberries

4 cinnamon sticks

1. In a small bowl, whisk together the orange juice and zest, lemon juice and zest, water, cloves, and syrup.

2. Place the cranberries and cinnamon sticks in the slow cooker. Pour the juice mixture over the cranberries, and toss to combine.

3. Cook on low for 4 hours.

4. Allow the sauce to slightly cool. Remove and discard cinnamon sticks.

5. Using a blender or immersion blender, blend the cranberry sauce until smooth. For a chunkier sauce, mash with the back of a fork.

TOBY'S TIP: Swap the maple syrup for your sweetener of choice, including unsulphured molasses or honey.

Serving size: ¼ cup
Per serving: Calories: 64; Total fat: 0g; Saturated fat: 0g; Protein: 0g; Carbohydrates: 17g; Fiber: 2g; Sodium: 3mg

Easy Mango Chutney

GLUTEN-FREE | DAIRY-FREE | VEGAN | VEGETARIAN

One of my favorite ways to enjoy chicken or fish is topped with mango chutney. However, I've never found jarred chutney that I loved nutritionally or with the flavor I wanted. So instead, I created this simple mango chutney that makes my taste buds dance for joy.

MAKES 2½ CUPS

Prep time: 15 minutes

Cook time: 30 minutes

3 mangos, peeled and diced

4 pitted dates, chopped

3 tablespoons white wine vinegar

Zest and juice of ½ lemon

3 garlic cloves, minced

2 tablespoons grated fresh ginger

⅛ teaspoon red pepper flakes

1. In a medium saucepan over medium heat, add the mango, dates, vinegar, lemon zest and juice, garlic, ginger, and red pepper flakes, stirring to combine. Bring the mixture to a boil. Reduce heat to low, cover, and simmer for 30 minutes, stirring occasionally.

2. Remove from heat and allow to cool for 10 minutes. Place the chutney in a blender, and blend until mostly smooth, but leaving some chunks.

3. Store covered in the refrigerator for up to 3 days.

TOBY'S TIP: Keep a bag of pitted dates in your pantry. Use them instead of sweeteners like sugar or honey in smoothies, chutney, and snack bites.

Serving size: ¼ cup

Per serving: Calories: 65; Total fat: 0g; Saturated fat: 0g; Protein: 1g; Carbohydrates: 17g; Fiber: 2g; Sodium: 2mg

Homemade Bread Crumbs

DAIRY-FREE | VEGAN | VEGETARIAN

In my kosher home growing up, my mother always bought special kosher bread crumbs. I never understood why, until one day I asked her. As it turns out, many store-bought varieties of flavored bread crumbs contain cheese to enhance the flavor. Since my mom used bread crumbs to bread chicken, she didn't want to combine the meat and the cheese (a no-no in a kosher house). Although I don't keep kosher, I still like to make my own bread crumbs so I can use them plain or flavored as I see fit.

MAKES 1½ CUPS

30-MINUTE

Prep time: 5 minutes
Cook time: 10 minutes

4 slices 100% whole-wheat bread

1. Preheat the oven to 350°F.

2. Tear the bread into bite-size pieces. Place in the food processor and pulse until reduced to fine crumbs, about 30 seconds.

3. Sprinkle the crumbs in a single layer on an ungreased baking sheet. Toast in the oven for 10 minutes, until slightly browned. Remove from the oven.

4. Using a wooden spoon, toss the bread crumbs, breaking up any clumps.

5. Store in a resealable container at room temperature for up to 1 week.

TOBY'S TIP: Always look for whole-wheat bread with 100% whole wheat listed as the first ingredient on the package.

Serving size: ¼ cup
Per serving: Calories: 73; Total fat: 1g; Saturated fat: 0g; Protein: 3g; Carbohydrates: 13g; Fiber: 2g; Sodium: 147mg

Homemade Caramel Sauce

GLUTEN-FREE | VEGETARIAN

Ever check the ingredient list of store-bought caramel sauce? It's a vast laundry list, including different forms of sugar, numerous colors, and additives. I prefer to make my own using ingredients from my pantry, and now you can, too!

MAKES 1 CUP

30-MINUTE

Prep time: 5 minutes

Cook time: 5 minutes

½ cup plus 2 tablespoons granulated sugar

4 tablespoons (½ stick) unsalted butter

6 tablespoons heavy (whipping) cream

1 teaspoon vanilla extract

¼ teaspoon salt

1. In a small saucepan over low heat, add the sugar and butter. Cook, stirring continuously, until the mixture turns a light brown color, about 4 minutes.

2. Add the heavy cream and stir. When the steam has dissipated, stir rapidly for about 1 minute to combine the mixture. Remove from heat, and stir in the vanilla and salt.

TOBY'S TIP: Use the caramel sauce as a dip for fruit, or top a spoonful over Greek yogurt.

Serving size: 1 tablespoon

Per serving: Calories: 75; Total fat: 5g; Saturated fat: 3g; Protein: 0g; Carbohydrates: 8g; Fiber: 0g; Sodium: 39mg

Vanilla-Infused Whipped Cream

When I was growing up, my grandma babysat me while my parents were at work. One of her favorite snacks to serve was strawberries with whipped cream. Mind you, it was the overly processed whipped topping you can find in the frozen section of the grocery store, which of course I loved at the time. But once I started dining out at good restaurants, my grown-up palate realized that freshly made whipped cream can taste more naturally sweet and creamy! That's when I started making my own, and now I use it for pies and trifles, and as a dip my fresh strawberries.

MAKES 2 CUPS

ONE POT/ONE PAN
30-MINUTE

Prep time: 10 minutes

1 cup heavy (whipping) cream

¼ cup granulated sugar

1 teaspoon vanilla extract

1. Using an electric hand mixer, whip the heavy cream until peaks form, about 5 minutes.

2. Add the sugar and vanilla, and continue whipping until well incorporated.

TOBY'S TIP: Instead of vanilla extract, try 1 tablespoon bourbon or 1 teaspoon ground cinnamon to infuse the whipped cream.

Serving size: 2 tablespoons
Per serving: Calories: 63; Total fat: 5g; Saturated fat: 4g; Protein: 0g; Carbohydrates: 4g; Fiber: 0g; Sodium: 5mg

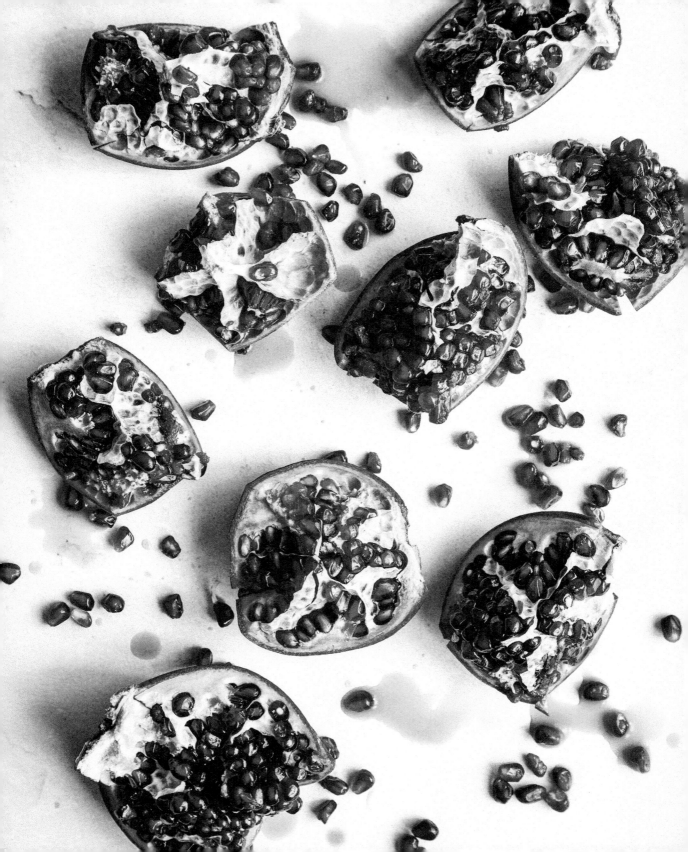

Measurements and Conversions

VOLUME EQUIVALENTS (LIQUID)

US STANDARD	US STANDARD (OUNCES)	METRIC (APPROXIMATE)
2 tablespoons	1 fl. oz.	30 mL
¼ cup	2 fl. oz.	60 mL
½ cup	4 fl. oz.	120 mL
1 cup	8 fl. oz.	240 mL
1½ cups	12 fl. oz.	355 mL
2 cups or 1 pint	16 fl. oz.	475 mL
4 cups or 1 quart	32 fl. oz.	1 L
1 gallon	128 fl. oz.	4 L

OVEN TEMPERATURES

FAHRENHEIT	CELSIUS (APPROXIMATE)
250°F	120°C
300°F	150°C
325°F	165°C
350°F	180°C
375°F	190°C
400°F	200°C
425°F	220°C
450°F	230°C

VOLUME EQUIVALENTS (DRY)

US STANDARD	METRIC (APPROXIMATE)
⅛ teaspoon	0.5 mL
¼ teaspoon	1 mL
½ teaspoon	2 mL
¾ teaspoon	4 mL
1 teaspoon	5 mL
1 tablespoon	15 mL
¼ cup	59 mL
⅓ cup	79 mL
½ cup	118 mL
⅔ cup	156 mL
¾ cup	177 mL
1 cup	235 mL
2 cups or 1 pint	475 mL
3 cups	700 mL
4 cups or 1 quart	1 L

WEIGHT EQUIVALENTS

US STANDARD	METRIC (APPROXIMATE)
½ ounce	15 g
1 ounce	30 g
2 ounces	60 g
4 ounces	115 g
8 ounces	225 g
12 ounces	340 g
16 ounces or 1 pound	455 g

References

Duyff, Roberta L. "Sodium Reduction in Canned Beans after Draining, Rinsing." *Journal of Culinary Science & Technology* 9, no. 2 (June 2011): 106–12. www.tandfonline.com/doi/abs/10.1080/15428052.2011.582405.

Freedman, Marjorie R., and Victor Fulgoli. "Canned Vegetable and Fruit Consumption Is Associated with Changes in Nutrient Intake and Higher Diet Quality in Children and Adults: National Health and Nutrition Examination Survey 2001–2010." *Journal of the Academy of Nutrition and Dietetics* 116, no. 6 (June 2016): 940–48. jandonline.org/article/S2212-2672%2815%2901587-7/abstract.

National Institutes of Health. "Aim for a Healthy Weight: Facts about a Healthy Weight." Accessed October 30, 2017. www.nhlbi.nih.gov/health/educational /lose_wt/index.htm.

U.S. Department of Agriculture. "Key Elements of Healthy Eating Patterns," in *Dietary Guidelines 2015–2020*. Accessed October 30, 2017. health.gov /dietaryguidelines/2015/guidelines/chapter-1/examples-of-other-healthy -eating-patterns/.

U.S. Department of Agriculture, Agricultural Research Service, Nutrient Data Laboratory. "USDA National Nutrient Database for Standard Reference, Release 28." September 2015, slightly revised May 2016. https://ndb.nal.usda.gov /ndb/search/list?ds=Standard+Reference.

U.S. Food and Drug Administration. "Qualified Claims About Cardiovascular Disease Risk: Nuts & Heart Disease." Docket No. 02P-0505. July 14, 2003. https://www.fda.gov/Food/LabelingNutrition/ucm073992.htm#cardio.

U.S. News & World Report. "Best Diet Rankings." Accessed October 30, 2017. health.usnews.com/best-diet/best-diets-overall.

Wallace, Taylor C., and Victor L. Fulgoni, III. "Assessment of Total Choline Intakes in the United States." *Journal of the American College of Nutrition* 35, no. 2 (2016): 108–12. www.ncbi.nlm.nih.gov/pubmed/26886842.

Recipe Type Index

Freezer-Friendly Recipes

Gluten-Free Recipes

One-Pot/One-Pan Recipes

Paleo-Friendly Recipes

Slow Cooker Recipes

30-Minute Recipes

Recipe Title Index

Index

Acknowledgments

There are many people I want to thank for making this cookbook possible. First and foremost, thank you to my three children, Schoen, Ellena, and Micah, for bearing with me through my insane schedule. Ellena and Micah, thank you for helping me test many of these recipes and for sitting with me for hours in the kitchen. Schoen, thank you for loving my food, especially my chicken Parm in this cookbook! All three of you are the forces that drive everything I do and have taught me the true meaning of life and love. Thank you to my parents for always supporting me. My dad, Henry Oksman, always taught me that anything is possible if you put your mind to it. I have found this advice true every time I achieve a milestone in my life. My mother, Zipporah Oksman, showed me what it is to truly be passionate about food and cooking. The bond we share in becoming registered dietitians together will be cherished forever. Finally, thank you to my loving boyfriend, Shaun Swersky, who is my ultimate taste tester. You have been there for me throughout this process, every step of the way.

A huge thank-you to my teammate and friend, Gail Watson, MS, who has dedicated her time and efforts to this project, and my assistant, Cristiane Camargo, for helping me with anything and everything that needed to get done.

Last but certainly not least, thank you to my literary agents Sally Ekus and Jaimee Constantine from the Lisa Ekus Group for your support and kindness throughout this process. Many thanks to my editor, Clara Song Lee, and Elizabeth Castoria from Callisto Media for bringing this project to life and being an absolute pleasure to work with.

About the Author

TOBY AMIDOR, MS, RD, CDN, a veteran in the food and nutrition industry with close to 20 years of experience, is a leading dietitian and recipe developer who believes that healthy and wholesome food can also be appetizing and delicious.

Toby is the founder of Toby Amidor Nutrition, where she provides nutrition and food safety consulting services for individuals, restaurants, and food brands. For 10 years, she has been the nutrition expert for FoodNetwork.com and founding contributor to FoodNetwork.com's *Healthy Eats* blog. She is a regular contributor to *U.S. News & World Report Eat + Run* blog and MensFitness.com, and she has her own "Ask the Expert" column in *Today's Dietitian* magazine. She also freelances for *Furthermore* from Equinox and SparkPeople.com, and has been quoted in publications like FoxNews.com, Self.com, *Oxygen Magazine*, *Dr. Oz The Good Life*, Mic.com, *Reader's Digest*, Shape.com, *Women's Health*, *Redbook*, *Men's Journal*, *Huffington Post*, *Everyday Health*, and more. Toby has also appeared on television, including *The Dr. Oz Show*, *AMHQ* with Sam Champion, Fox 5 NY's *Good Day Street Talk*, and *San Antonio Live*. For the past eight years, she has been an adjunct professor at Teachers College, Columbia University, and is currently an adjunct professor at Hunter College School of Urban Public Health in New York City.

Toby trained as a clinical dietitian at New York University. Previously, she was a consultant on Bobby Deen's cooking show, *Not My Mama's Meals*. Through ongoing consulting and faculty positions, she has established herself as one of the top experts in culinary nutrition, food safety, and nutrition communication.

Learn more about Toby on her website, TobyAmidorNutrition.com.

CPSIA information can be obtained
at www.ICGtesting.com
Printed in the USA
BVOW11s0059090318
509612BV00001B/1/P